CAREFUL EATING: BODIES, FOOD AND CARE

How wonderful, frightening or both for someone to take the care to make sure we eat properly, an interaction potentiated with both love and power! This engaging and diverse collection beautifully shows how – whether in families, clinics, schools or many other contexts – there is much more to the intimacies created through food than one may often imagine and sometimes more than we might care to think about.

Jon Holtzman, Western Michigan University, USA

T0298665

Critical Food Studies

Series Editor
Michael K. Goodman, Kings College London, UK

The study of food has seldom been more pressing or prescient. From the intensifying globalization of food, a world-wide food crisis and the continuing inequalities of its production and consumption, to food's exploding media presence, and its growing re-connections to places and people through 'alternative food movements', this series promotes critical explorations of contemporary food cultures and politics. Building on previous but disparate scholarship, its overall aims are to develop innovative and theoretical lenses and empirical material in order to contribute to – but also begin to more fully delineate – the confines and confluences of an agenda of critical food research and writing.

Of particular concern are original theoretical and empirical treatments of the materializations of food politics, meanings and representations, the shifting political economies and ecologies of food production and consumption and the growing transgressions between alternative and corporatist food networks.

Other titles in the series include:

Food Transgressions
Making Sense of Contemporary Food Politics
Edited by Michael K. Goodman and Colin Sage
9780754679707

Doing Nutrition Differently
Critical Approaches to Diet and Dietary Intervention
Edited by Allison Hayes-Conroy and Jessica Hayes-Conroy
9781409434795

Geographies of Race and Food
Fields, Bodies, Markets
Edited by Rachel Slocum and Arun Saldanha
9781409469254

Why We Eat, How We Eat
Edited by Emma-Jayne Abbots and Anna Lavis
9781409447252

Careful Eating: Bodies, Food and Care

Edited by

EMMA-JAYNE ABBOTS
*University of Wales Trinity Saint David and
SOAS, University of London, UK*

ANNA LAVIS
*University of Birmingham
and University of Oxford, UK*

LUCI ATTALA
*University of Wales Trinity Saint David
and Open University, UK*

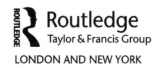

Routledge
Taylor & Francis Group

LONDON AND NEW YORK

First published 2015 by Ashgate Publishing

Published 2016 by Routledge
2 Park Square, Milton Park, Abingdon, Oxon OX14 4RN
711 Third Avenue, New York, NY 10017, USA

First issued in paperback 2017

Routledge is an imprint of the Taylor & Francis Group, an informa business

British Library Cataloguing in Publication Data
A catalogue record for this book is available from the British Library

The Library of Congress has been applied for

ISBN 13: 978-1-138-30847-3 (pbk)
ISBN 13: 978-1-4723-3948-2 (hbk)

Contents

Notes on Editors and Contributors

Editors

Emma-Jayne Abbots is a Senior Lecturer in Anthropology and Heritage at the University of Wales Trinity Saint David and a Research Associate at the SOAS Food Studies Centre, University of London. Her research focuses on the cultural politics of food and the visceral, material and embodied practices of its production, preparation, distribution and consumption: she is broadly concerned with the (re)production and mediation of knowledge and the political and environmental ecologies in which knowledge-making takes place. She has further related interests in: food and migration; heritage foods; the media; domestic labour relations; gender and class dynamics; and kinship, care and intimacies. In addition to a range of articles and chapters on these topics, Abbots is the co-editor with Anna Lavis of *Why We Eat, How We Eat: Contemporary Encounters between Foods and Bodies* (Ashgate, 2013) and is currently preparing a book entitled *The Agency of Eating: Mediation, Food and the Body* (Bloomsbury).

Anna Lavis is a medical anthropologist whose research focuses on embodied intimacies of illness and caregiving, particularly in relation to mental health and with an emphasis on gender and young people. As a Research Fellow at the University of Birmingham, she leads studies into lived experiences of psychosis and eating disorders . Anna has written about (not) eating and food more widely, critically interrogating eating across various empirical contexts as well as exploring (im)materialities of food and bodies. She co-edited *Why We Eat, How We Eat: Contemporary Encounters between Foods and Bodies* (Ashgate, 2013) with Emma-Jayne Abbots. She is also an honorary Research Associate in the Institute of Social and Cultural Anthropology, University of Oxford. There, with Karin Eli, she founded the *Body and Being Network*, a research initiative that creates public events by developing interdisciplinary dialogues about the body between social and medical scientists and performance artists.

Luci Attala is a Lecturer in Anthropology at University of Wales, Trinity Saint David and Associate Lecturer in Health and Social Care with the Open University. Her research interests are underpinned by a focus on materialities with specific attention afforded to the coalescing themes of incorporation, ingestion and the becomings of eco-logical bodies as produced by the ingestive relationships interacting bodies/subjects create. Luci is currently completing a PhD at Exeter University that explores engagements with water by a reforestation initiative in rural Kenya and considers water's part in organizing human bodies and social behaviours in different settings. Taking inspiration from post-humanism, the more-than-human move and multispecies ethnographies, her work maps the flows of water through various bodies (including botanical ones) and thus also reconsiders orthodox understandings of plant–human interactions within the body and within other/wider environmental settings.

Notes on Contributors

Benjamin Coles is a Lecturer in Political and Economic Geography at the University of Leicester. His research interests centre on place, space and scale, with a particular interest in the relationship(s) between place-making, commodity culture and the production and consumption of food. He has explored these interests in a number of diverse ethnographic settings from chicken production in Brazil to coffee drinking in London's Borough Market.

Karin Eli is a postdoctoral researcher at the University of Oxford's Institute of Social and Cultural Anthropology, where her research projects focus on the subjective experience of eating disorders, and on consumer engagement with food governance. She has conducted extensive narrative-based fieldwork research on eating disorders in Israel and the UK, and is co-editor of *Obesity, Eating Disorders and the Media* (Ashgate, 2014). Karin is a member of the Unit of Biocultural Variation and Obesity and of the Oxford Martin Programme on the Future of Food, both at the University of Oxford.

Rick Flowers is a convenor of a research program about Everyday, Cultural and Public Pedagogies at the University of Technology, Sydney, which is currently undertaking research about food pedagogies and organizing for multiculturalism in various tourism projects, including ethnic food tours and multicultural festivals. He is currently editing a book for the Ashgate critical food series called *Food Pedagogies* with Elaine Swan. Their work draws on Elaine's interests in critical race and feminist perspectives, and Rick's interests in popular education and social action.

Mike Goodman is a Professor of Geography in the Geography and Environmental Science Department, Reading University. Recent publications include *Alternative Food Networks* with David Goodman and Melanie DuPuis (Routledge, 2012) and *Food Transgressions: Making Sense of Contemporary Food Politics* (Ashgate, 2014 with Colin Sage). He edits the Critical Food Studies book series for Ashgate and the Contemporary Food Studies book series for Bloomsbury. Forthcoming publications include a special issue of *Geoforum* (with Josee Johnston) on food, media and space, a second in *Food, Culture and Society* (also with Josee

Johnston) on celebrity and spectacular food politics, and a third in *Environmental Communications* on the cultural politics of media and environment.

Michelle Jones works in the Office of the Chief Public Health Officer, *SA Health*. Michelle has managed the evaluations of childhood obesity prevention programs; and men's sex, violent offender and Aboriginal treatment programs. Her PhD examined discourses of domestic violence. Michelle's research interests include public health, program evaluation, social justice and equity, Aboriginal health, women's health and men's violence against women.

Antje Lindenmeyer is a Lecturer in Qualitative Methods in the Department of Primary Care Clinical Sciences at the University of Birmingham. Her background is in social sciences and her research interests centre on human interaction and understanding around health and illness, including the experience of living with illness and the social context of healthcare encounters. As part of this, she is very interested in social interactions around food in everyday life and intersections between these interactions and discourses around health promotion.

Amy K. McLennan is an Early Career Teaching and Research Fellow in Medical Anthropology at the University of Oxford. She has a dual background in the medical and social sciences, and has previously carried out long-term ethnographic fieldwork in Oceania. Her research is currently focused on historical socio-political change, food habits, and demographic health change. She is particularly interested in developing interdisciplinary approaches to better understand and address obesity and nutrition-related non-communicable diseases.

Vivienne Moore is a social epidemiologist with scholarly interests in the social determinants of health, including gender roles and relations, and life course epidemiology. She is noted for fostering and engaging in multi-disciplinary research. She has published over 70 peer-reviewed journal articles and book chapters.

Signe Rousseau teaches critical literacy at the University of Cape Town, where she also completed her doctoral and post-doctoral work. She is the author of *Food Media: Celebrity Chefs and the Politics of Everyday Interference* (2012), and *Food and Social Media: You Are What You Tweet* (2012), and a contributing author to *The Business of Food: Encyclopedia of the Food and Drink Industries* (2008), *Food Cultures of the World* (2011), *Icons of American Cooking* (2011), *The Oxford Encyclopedia of American Food and Drink* (2012), and *A Cultural History of Food, The Modern Age (1920-2000)* (2012).

Tanja Schneider is a Research Fellow in Science and Technology Studies at the Institute for Science, Innovation and Society and the Saïd Business School, University of Oxford. Her research focuses on market(ing) and governing practices, specifically in relation to food. Her most recent publications address the governance of genetically modified and functional foods in Europe, the emergence of restless forms of consumer behaviour in the food system and the marketing of health food and healthy eating practices in Australia and Europe. Tanja is also a Fellow of the Unit of Biocultural Variation and Obesity and of the Oxford Martin Programme on the Future of Food, both at the University of Oxford.

Elaine Swan is a convenor of a research program about Everyday, Cultural and Public Pedagogies at the University of Technology Sydney, along with Rick Flowers. They are currently undertaking research about food pedagogies and multiculturalism in various tourism projects, including ethnic food tours and multicultural festivals. They are currently editing a book for the Ashgate critical food series called *Food Pedagogies*. Their work draws on Elaine's interests in critical race and feminist perspectives, and Rick's interests in popular education and social action.

José Teixeira graduated in Sociology from the ISCTE-IUL (Lisbon University Institute) in 2010. He is currently conducting the final dissertation for a Masters on Communication, Culture and Information Technology (ISCTE-IUL), about the eating habits of families with children. He has worked as a Research Assistant on the project *Between the School and the Family: Children's Food Knowledge and Eating Practices* (FCT/Ministry of Science and Technology, Portugal) since June 2011.

Mónica Truninger is a Senior Research Fellow at the Institute of Social Sciences (University of Lisbon, Portugal) and visiting research fellow at the Sustainable Consumption Institute (University of Manchester, UK). Her main research interests include school meals and children's eating habits, domestic technologies and cooking practices, sustainable consumption and provisioning systems. She is Principal Investigator of a research project on school meals and children's food knowledge and practices (FCT/Ministry of Science and Technology, Portugal). She has published in national and international peer-review journals (e.g. *Journal of Consumer Culture*; *Trends in Food Science and Technology*). Recent books include *O Campo Vem à Cidade: Agricultura Biológica, Mercado e Consumo Sustentável* (Lisbon: ICS Press, 2010) [The countryside comes to the city: organic farming, market and sustainable consumption].

Paul Ward is the Head of the Discipline of Public Health and Associate Dean (Research), at the Faculty of Medicine, Nursing and Health Sciences, Flinders University, Australia. Paul is a social scientist with research interests around lay and professional perceptions, knowledge and understandings of health, healthcare, risk, resilience and trust.

Megan Warin is a Social Anthropologist and Australian Research Council Future Fellow in the Discipline of Gender Studies and Social Analysis at the University of Adelaide, Australia. Her current research interests span theories of embodiment and sensory aesthetics, intersections of class and gender in experiences of obesity, public understanding of obesity science, the anthropology of epigentics and desire and denial in eating disorders.

Tanya Zivkovic is a Social Anthropologist whose research explores the body and cultural trajectories of the life course. Tanya's research interests include work on death, relics, and reincarnation among Tibetan Buddhist lamas, 'the child', gender and obesity, and more recently Tibetan healing and biomedicine. Tanya is a Senior Research Fellow in the Discipline of Gender Studies and Social Analysis, University of Adelaide, and her book *Death and Reincarnation in Tibetan Buddhism* was published by Routledge in 2014.

Acknowledgements

First and foremost we should like to express our gratitude to all the authors who have contributed to this volume. Your willingness to engage with the theme, your openness to critiques and suggestions, and your ability to bear tight deadlines has been second to none, and it has been a pleasure to work with you all.

Our thanks also go to our series editor, Mike Goodman, for his constant enthusiasm and support for our projects, as well as for the thought-provoking discussions and insightful comments.

At Ashgate, our commissioning editor, Katy Crossan, is always a joy to work with. Our appreciation also goes to Carolyn Court, Margaret Younger, and our editor Philip Stirups for seeing this volume through the production process.

Thanks are also due to Eloise Govier for her beautiful cover art and to the anonymous reviewer for their positive and constructive feedback.

We are fortunate to have a number of colleagues and friends who are engaging with similar academic questions to ours, and who have inevitably informed the ways we approach the critical study of food, caregiving, and the embodied entanglements between eating and caring. Our appreciation, in particular, goes to Ben Coles, Karin Eli, Linda Everard, Rachel Foskett-Tharby, Jakob A. Klein, Antje Lindenmeyer, Amy McLennan, Anne Murcott, Louise Steel, Stanley Ulijaszek, Harry G. West and Katharina Zinn.

Finally, Emma-Jayne Abbots would personally like to thank her co-editors, Anna and Luci, not only for their intellectual inspiration and friendship, but also for their commitment and enthusiasm – both to this project and those that lie beyond. Thanks also to David Abbots, for his patience, his humour and his tendency to ask the awkward questions.

Anna Lavis would like to acknowledge the inspiring collaboration and friendship of Emma-Jayne and Luci; working with you on this has been a pleasure. My gratitude also goes to Pamela and David Lavis for their support, in all its varied forms, both during the production of this book and beyond its pages. Finally, thank you to David Martin for being his brilliant self.

And in genuine appreciation of their support, encouragement and guidance on what has been, for her, a steep learning curve, Luci Attala would also like to offer warm and sincere heart-felt thanks to her co-editors Emma-Jayne and Anna – working with these two whirlwinds has been both an honour and an invaluable education. In addition, she thanks her four beautiful children for inspiring her (despite all their nonsense), and finally, thanks to Ru Hartwell for being a rock, and a constantly sanguine and patient listener throughout.

Introduction

Reflecting on the Embodied Intersections
of Eating and Caring

Anna Lavis, Emma-Jayne Abbots and Luci Attala

The aim of *Careful Eating* is to critically reflect on the many and varied relationships between food and care. Specifically, it investigates how these relationships are mobilized to shape and intervene in individual bodies, as well as how they may be both enacted and resisted in and through those bodies. It thereby develops current critical debates regarding how care, in the context of food and eating, may so often be a political mechanism through which the self and the Other are (re)produced and social hierarchies constructed. As such, this transdisciplinary volume draws into dialogue diverse ways of addressing a currently neglected, yet critically important, question regarding the ways in which eating and caring interact on multiple scales: From state-led interventions and public health discourses to the workplace, from the market to the home, and in the intimacies of individual eating and feeding practices. Engaging with the often-jagged political intersections of food and care across these scales, and paying attention to the bodies caught up in them, offers new ways of thinking through urgent contemporary concerns regarding food and social justice. It addresses fundamental questions regarding how, as human beings, we care (or not) for and about ourselves and Others, our communities and environments. This involves drawing attention to the terms 'caring' and 'eating' themselves, asking what each is, what relationships they create and rupture, and how their interplays are experienced in everyday life. By taking account of these multi-directional flows of engagement between eating and caring practices, the volume's contributors elucidate: how eating practices mobilize discourses and forms of care; how discourses and practices of care (look to) shape particular forms of eating and food preferences; and how it is often in the bodies of individual consumers that eating and caring encounter one another. These three central theoretical dimensions are the organizing principles around which the chapters' diverse perspectives coalesce, and the volume is constructed.

Eating and caring are inherently bound together. Normatively framed as simultaneously instinctive and didactic, both are understood as something we do and something we learn to do in order to reproduce and sustain social and biological life. It has been suggested that, just as multiple roles are assumed in relation to food throughout the lifecourse, with individuals feeding Others as well as eating, 'what most people spend their lives doing [is] caring for themselves, for others, and for the world' (Tronto 1993: x). Yet although individuals' care practices are often relational and intimate like their food choices, they can also be socially prescribed, constrained and even enforced. As such, whilst recognizing the central importance of caregiving practices to human life and society, we suggest that care is also not necessarily as benign as it might appear. Mirroring recent understandings of the tensions and power dynamics embedded in both the production and consumption of food (Abbots and Lavis 2013; Holtzman 2013), caring has been shown to be heavy with moral value and is often entangled in culturally-embedded notions of the 'right' and the 'good' (Barnes 2012; Gilligan 1982). Commodified as well as given, both food and care practices are arguably as political as they are moral (Tronto 1993). Eating and caring can therefore be further understood not only as performances of reproduction, but also of production: ones that constitute Others and (re)establish relations between those Others and selves. *Careful Eating* argues that it is the myriad and diverging ways in which care is defined and utilized that underpin this production. This slippery multiplicity is central to care's political malleability within contemporary social and cultural debates around food; it allows the seemingly benign concept of care to be mobilized and used to produce highly politicized knowledge claims about eating that intervene in, constrain and reshape individual bodies and their everyday practices of consumption. Such claims, in turn, also construct eating and feeding as caring or care-less acts – by the self, for the self and for Others. As such, just as there are many points of contact between eating and caring at the level of political agendas and cultural discourses, they also meet in the biological and subjective depths of the body. Viscerally illustrating what has been termed 'the corporeality of the social and the sociality of corporeality' (Blackman 2008: 3), both eating and caring are profoundly social practices to which the body is central. Mirroring the way in which particular bodies are produced, denigrated or caught up in (bio)political framings of food, both eating and caring are intrinsically embodied performances; political relations and cultural imaginings may be resisted and disrupted by, as well as played out in, individual eating bodies.

Highlighting this circulation and ingestion of knowledge claims engenders a question that is central this volume: Why and how do individuals, groups, institutions and agencies care about what Others eat? And, secondly, what forms of sociality and social bodies are made and negotiated, ruptured and ignored, or rendered visible and invisible, in these encounters between individual eating bodies and the caring agendas of Others? This volume illustrates that there are no easy answers to these questions. There is, rather, a range of responses and reactions and these pose further nuanced and reflexive questions across a variety of contexts and disciplines: In what ways do discourses of 'good' and 'proper' food and eating utilize the concept of care to promote their ideologies? How is care manipulated to alter the eating practices of others? How is care for the social body used to govern and regulate individual bodies? How do individuals respond to such governance? How do individuals demonstrate their care for and about Others by eating as well as feeding? How is agency dispersed along the networks that are created by food and eating practices, and how does this contrast to the conceptualizations of agency embedded in notions of care? To explore these questions and others, the individual chapters of this volume are drawn from anthropology; geography; cultural studies; primary health care; public health; gender studies; critical literacy; science and technology studies; education and sociology. Although diverse in approach, each contributor starts from the premise that eating and caring are simultaneously individual and social, material and symbolic, ideological and political, and all have been challenged to explore the multi-dimensionality of the interplays and entanglements between eating and caring. Together the contributors offer a unique and creative pathway into issues as diverse as body size and eating disorders; children's dietary guidelines; inequality and poverty; mass and social media; ethical eating; ecological and cultural sustainability; food tourism; and the cultural politics of contemporary food systems.

The purpose of this collection then is to forge interdisciplinary and dialogic (see Bakhtin 1982) ways in which to 'strip back' the discourses of care that we suggest perpetually frame the eating practices of Others, and reveal the (re)production of embodied power dynamics that are inherent, but commonly obscured, in such discourses. The contributors elucidate the many socio-material relationalities of eating and caring, illustrating these to be both political and politicized. Through their empirically-grounded richness and theoretical complexity, the chapters trace the often-hidden ways in which eating and caring may (be made to) isolate and divide as much as create sociality and cohesion. It is in this insight that the central theoretical contribution of the volume as a whole lies; it demonstrates how paying attention to eating and caring offers up a new critical lens onto broader contemporary questions regarding food, (bio)politics and social justice. By drawing attention to these political processes across such a diverse range of contexts, the chapters elucidate the ways in which individual eating bodies are both knowingly and unknowingly entangled in, and made by, circulating notions of care.

As such, *Careful Eating* extends and productively reverses the focus of our earlier volume in this series, entitled *Why We Eat, How We Eat* (Abbots and Lavis 2013). That volume explored the ways in which Others – bodies, agents, institutions and nations – are performed and produced through the act of eating, as webs of relations flow outwards from the individual eater. Maintaining the focus on eating initiated there, this volume now explores not only how imaginings, mobilizations and relationships of care actively shape eating, but also the part played by eating in the production and breaching of performances of care. By paying attention to this multi-directionality of entanglements between food and care, *Careful Eating* examines what is made and unmade by the individual act of eating itself, and also the ways in which eating is viewed, critiqued and governed by Others. In so doing, we retain the focus on food both inside and outside of bodies initially presented in *Why We Eat, How We Eat*, but now turn to develop this by reflecting on how individual eating bodies are lived, shaped and sculpted by and through care, and how care is ingested, felt and lived in the 'ordinary' (Stewart 2007) spaces of everyday lives.

Careful Eating is organized into three parts that mirror the three central theoretical dimensions of the volume noted above. Within each part, we have purposefully juxtaposed chapters with differing approaches and disciplinary backgrounds in order to create dialogue through which each may illuminate the others. Part I, comprising chapters by Flowers and Swan, Rousseau, and Abbots, traces how eating performs relationships of care. It examines how particular food practices and preferences are framed as enacting care more than others and shows how specific foods, in turn, come to be valued as care-full, while others are constructed as care-less. In so doing, this part elucidates ways in which these subjective valorizations are informed by, and reproduce, political dynamics and how relations of otherness may be created through proximity as much as distance. In Part II, Lavis, Zivkovik et al. and Lindenmeyer all explore bodies as the primary sites in which caring and eating encounter one another in everyday life. Each, in a different way, captures the multi-directionality and myriad scales of this encounter, demonstrating that in individual moments of eating and feeding, care may not always be felt to be so 'caring', or food so 'good' or 'right'. Part III reverses the flow of Part I and directs attention to the ways in which discourses of care perform eating. Here, Coles, Eli et al., and Truninger and Teixeira focus on how political and ideological modes of caring frame eating behaviours, and illustrate, in turn, how care is simultaneously placed and enacted. In so doing, the chapters in this part deconstruct how social and personal frameworks embedded in caring actions shape eating practices.

Disentangling the Entanglements between Eating and Caring

The chapters of this volume all demonstrate that care is a foundational concept in current critical debates about 'good' and 'proper' eating across a range of contexts, including clinical settings, schools and public institutions, retailers and the market, and online forums. Yet a systematic critical analysis of the concept of care in relation to food practices and preferences has, to date, been largely absent from the interdisciplinary field of Food Studies. It has been commonly implied – although not explicitly drawn out as a concept worthy of examination – in a wide range of accounts of food selection and preparation, feeding and eating. It is this body of work that provides, in part, the ethnographic and theoretical foundations of our approach and which we look to extend here by drawing care explicitly to the fore for closer interrogation.

Current scholarship within Food Studies has often invoked a definition of care in a soft, virtuous form, associating it with commensality, affection, love, kinship and social cohesion. Caring what other people eat in these contexts, the literature tells us, is related to the forming of social bonds; it is a gesture of love and affection, a symbol of nurture, and the manner through which individuals are incorporated – culturally, emotionally and biologically – into a social group (Carsten 1997; Fischler 1988). Care manifests, then, in work that explores the interplays between food, being and belonging, and elucidates how feeding and eating are pivots around which identities, of both selves and groups, are forged and performed (Abbots 2011; Klein and Murcott 2014). This process is thrown into particularly sharp relief when senses of belonging are put into a state of flux or drawn into dialogue with those of Others, as in the context of migration and multiculturalism. Ray's (2004) study of middle class Bengali-Americans, for example, demonstrates how commensal sociality reproduces social relations between families and helps maintain cultural continuities. Renne (2007) highlights how attentiveness to what is eaten reinforces West African identity and community in the USA. Likewise, Toumainen (2011) points to the ways in which solidarity is fostered, and previously entrenched ethnic boundaries dissolved, among Ghanian migrants in London through shared food practices and preferences. The notion of 'culinary safe havens' (Saber and Posner 2013: 198) thus emerges in which eating is treated as a process through which intimacies are forged, boundaries blurred, coterminous bodies constituted and, as such, care enacted.

The Slipperiness of Care

In order to extend reflections on care within Food Studies beyond this softer conceptualization of caring, it is necessary to ask what caring is and what it means. To avoid the risk of not looking beyond the benign, even essential, life-sustaining aspects of care, we need to consider what else care might be and how it is conceived, provoked, inherited, mobilized, performed and rejected. Therefore, in addition to Food Studies literature, *Careful Eating* engages with the interdisciplinary body of literature that reflects on care. Thinking through care is a slippery exercise not only because care is diversely experienced, conceived of and applied to food and eating, but also because what 'to care' means is widely contested, with the opacity of the term extensively examined. A prominent example of such explorations is Finch and Grove's (1983) collection of essays entitled *A Labour of Love,* which explores and illustrates that caring is variously applied; to care may denote a feeling, a relationship or form of work (see also Fisher and Tonto 1990). Ungerson (1983) further bifurcates care into two converging manners of caring: care-for and care-about, a deconstruction that has helped to establish care as something one can do and something one can feel (Thomas 1993). In her more recent exploration Ungerson (2005) further elucidates that these dynamics of care as action, labour and performance as well as emotion, sentiment and feeling are still very much active with regards to how care is understood and delivered.

With some degree of agreement, Hinchliffe (2007) argues that when nurturing behaviours (and attitudes) are operating, care is signified. This frames caring as a manner of relating that is rooted in beneficence. As such, one can be said to care when one cultivates, cherishes, offers philanthropic or charitable support, or sustains attention to, an Other (be that a person, object, idea or place). It is this model of care that is particularly explored by Mol et al. (2010a. See also Mol 2008) who seek to draw the hidden embodied specificities of care work to attention, illustrating how care practices challenge rationalist notions of a bounded human. Instead, the authors suggest, they constitute and reveal 'the relations in which we make each other be' (Mol et al. 2010b: 15). This portrayal of care as a nourishing force makes it easy to believe that when care manifests 'good intentions' (Mol et al. 2010b: 12) prevail, and a 'good' is mobilized and produced. It is viewing care within this framework that enables it to assume the qualities of a virtue (see also Barnes 2006, 2012).

This supposition that care acts as a beneficent force draws much strength from the series of ethical philosophies that explore the concept of care with a view to ascribe value to personal, political and global caring, and to ultimately inspire a universally applicable 'ethic of care'. This could be seen as a social substrate from which emerge practices that support social justice and equality (see Barnes 2012; Held 2006; Tronto 1993). Wishing to illuminate how caregiving practices may underpin human society, scholars of an ethic of care propound this recognition to fashion *how* (not *if*) citizens care for each other. In turn, this framework has been utilized to disseminate models of best practice in a bid to promote and elucidate the hows of effective care (Twigg and Atkin 1994; Twigg 2006). Care emerges from this body of literature as at the root of our humanity and instrumental to mobilizing sociality (and thus survival), but it is simultaneously and paradoxically deemed flawed. As such, caring is legitimately re-appropriated and transformed into a set of skills and behaviours one can learn and become proficient in (Kubiak et al. 2007; Qureshi and Walker 1989). This slippage from instinct to learning allows discussion not only of how to teach the population to care, but also how to care 'correctly'. Care, thus, emerges as a troubled hybrid, conceptualized both as an innate ability and as a biopolitical force that governs and disciplines. It is framed as something persons instinctively do and yet as a process to be learnt that demands expert knowledge, guidance and training. As such, care manifests as an 'ontopolitical' force (Connolly 1995: 2) – a set of ideas that functions to 'fix possibilities, distribute explanatory elements, generate parameters within which an ethic is generated, and center (or decenter) assessments of identity, legitimacy, and responsibility' (ibid.: 2).

It can be argued, thus, that calls for an ethic of care conflate being caring (as a state) with the construction of a social framework of common and collective good. Such a conflation avoids the prickly issues of normativity, control and hierarchy that the implementation of a framework for caring is arguably liable to create (Foucault 1978). Additionally, these discussions nimbly sidestep explorations of the vast array of motivations attached to the multiplicities of being caring and, as such, avoid questions that might work to problematize what care is and does. This volume engages with, and challenges, these perspectives in order to interrogate how assumptions of care as a virtue may influence, pervade, and sculpt social and individual practices and discourses around food and eating. Furthermore, actions that claim to be rooted in care also produce numerous behaviours, conclusions and responses that may not be experienced as caring or care-full by all parties. Consequently, reflecting on caring *about* what Others eat – and perhaps, caring *for* Others through that concern – raise questions regarding how the taken-for-granted moral, righteous and worthy character of care allows demands to be made on social and individual (eating) behaviours. Thus what it means to care – that is to care-for, to care-about, to be caring – it seems, may not always be as caring as it appears, after all.

Regulated and Resistant Eating Bodies

By offering diverging examples of how caring is enacted and experienced both around and through eating, the following chapters demonstrate how the seeming benevolence of care is deeply embedded in governing processes of normativity, regulation and control. This recognition shifts the meaning of caring into a disposition or practice that is more than simply virtuous; it transforms into a mechanism of achieving outcomes that is at once wrapped in virtue but is also political. Accordingly, this volume traces how, when associated with food and eating, care may be problematically entwined around regulatory ideas of good or normative practices, citizens and bodies.

The ingesting bodies (of Others) have increasingly become key sites both of 'surveillance medicine' (Armstrong 1995. See also Foucault 2003) and of 'biopower', defined as the 'numerous and diverse techniques for achieving the subjugation of bodies and the control of populations' (Foucault 1978: 140) undertaken by nation states. In such a formulation, caring what Others eat and are fed emerges as a mode of discipline that is not only imposed upon individual bodies but also lived through these, as bodies are invested with technologies of power that render them docile (Foucault 1977). In this volume, this is highlighted by Truninger and Teixera, through their exploration of school meals as 'biopedagogies' (Wright and Harwood 2009). Abbots also shows this by examining the ways in which the governing classes in Highland Ecuador establish social distance in their attempts to discipline the eating behaviours, and shape the bodies, of the peasantry by subjectively constructing some forms of eating as care-full and others as care-less.

Within public health, the body has an extensive history as a site of such cultural and political disciplining around food. Public health in Britain, for example, has long emphasized structural factors that undermine wellbeing as well as bodily integrity and longevity. It has sought to intervene in these at the level of state policy (Twigg 2006. See also Lewis et al. 2000; Petersen and Lupton 1996), with food featuring in these processes since the nineteenth century (Baggott 2000). Underpinning much of those earlier interventionist policies were concerns over potential food shortages and malnutrition (Mills 1992). Underfed bodies were framed as both individually vulnerable and detrimental to the workforce, with a lack of food thereby regarded as potentially destabilizing to the individual and social body. Food insecurity and poverty, and their intersections with social justice, and indeed injustice, continue to be pressing issues, both in the global south and, as shown by the rise in food banks (Trussell Trust 2014), in the global north. Malnutrition in ageing populations, particularly in relation to dementia as well as poverty, is also a growing global concern (Donini et al. 2013; Pierson 1999). However, the bodies that are arguably framed as most in need of discipline in cultural imaginings and media discussions, especially in the global north, are those framed as 'obese'.

Caring about what Others eat has, perhaps, taken its most explicit public form in relation to the politics of what the WHO has controversially termed a 'global epidemic' (WHO 2000) of obesity. As Zivkovik et al. and Lindenmeyer explore in this volume, obesity has been the focus of many and varied public health initiatives and interventions. Since the advent of the 21st century, these have also underpinned a swathe of obesity-focused entertainment television, particularly in the UK and USA. This has arguably enabled such knowledge claims not only to travel, but also to be performed and accepted as 'fact' in ways that visually categorize and stigmatize Others' bodies (Eli and Lavis 2014; Inthorn and Boyce 2010; Oullette and Hay 2008). As Lindenmeyer's chapter shows, obesity-focused discussions of eating often draw a linear acultural relationship between food and body fat, which is contested (Aphramor et al. 2013). They also frame corporeal fat simply as excess without meaning, which has been challenged by explorations of its embodiment and materiality (Colls 2012; Lavis 2014; Murray 2005). Through such discourses, the body emerges as central to the enactment of neoliberal citizenship; eating and food preferences are thereby positioned as integral to a seemingly virtuous self-care that enacts 'good' citizenship through responsibilized caring for both the individual and social body. Eating becomes entangled in neoliberal notions of individual responsibility, and continuous self-improvement (Guthman 2011; Walkerdine 2003) with the feeding of Others, especially children, also an act that must be performed within disciplined parameters (Bell et al. 2009; Zivkovik et al. 2010). This latter, and its widespread gendering, is also particularly demonstrated in a slightly different but related context by debates around breastfeeding (see Faircloth 2010; Stearns 1999). Relationships between foods and bodies are therefore key ways in which 'technologies of the self' (Foucault 1988) are inculcated and enacted (see also Lupton 1996, 1997). As such, however, certain bodies and persons can also find themselves omitted from constructions of a 'good' citizen.

As care sits so awkwardly between the personal and the political, when offered to those considered at risk or vulnerable it can produce discomfort and resistance. This has been seen more widely in relation, particularly, to disability (Campbell and Oliver 1996) and mental health (Crossley and Crossley 2001), which have both seen important challenges to taken-for-granted paradigms of illness and care in recent years. These have sought to extend inclusion by exploring notions of citizenship and wellbeing, and have also highlighted individuals' agency and embeddedness in wider networks of relations as caregivers as well as receivers (see also Twigg 2006). In this volume, the potentially uncomfortable dynamics of care are drawn out by both Lindenmeyer's and Lavis' accounts of intimate interactions within clinical encounters. Lindenmeyer shows that the series of positions and identities created by care services do not only function as top-down models of intervention, but also work to affect all of those involved in the process. She thereby illustrates how experts, whilst enabled and authorized to convey proclamations on the how, when and what of caring practice generally, are also party to and instrumental in the production of new tensions, which emerge from the manner through which caring relationships are structured. As such, as Lavis explores, both carers and those being cared for negotiate between normative notions of care and the complexities and experiences of personal lived realities, from which alternative models of caring may emerge. Both of these chapters consequently not only point to the implicit power dynamics inveigled in caring, but also highlight that being cared for is not necessarily experienced as a positive intervention. They thereby demonstrate how care may become absent to itself in dialogues around food, as interventions that are wrapped up as care in the giving may not be experienced as care in the receiving.

Practices of resistance to such biopolitical, and indeed often biomedical, framings of the relationships between foods, care and individuals are also present in Abbots' account of discourses of good and proper eating propounded by the governing classes that define the preferred foods of the peasantry as lacking in care. Measures are consequently taken to encourage more careful eating practices which, Abbots shows, have little effect, with the peasantry enacting care for and through food in their own, more intimate ways, while continuing to consume those foods deemed care-less in public spaces. Likewise, Zivkovic et al.'s chapter explores how 'sweetness', in the form of refined sugars, is constructed in diverging ways by public health initiatives and individual eating bodies. Their ethnographically-rich discussion reveals how ingesting sugar in a context of social disadvantage contrasts to normative notions of a 'correct' diet; sweetness, they argue, 'emerges as a strategy of caring', which reclaims sugar from public health discourse, not only repositioning its categorization but also its materiality. As such, this chapter elucidates not only how seemingly well-meaning interventions concerned with the health of biological and social bodies can be regarded – and experienced – as an instrument of (attempted) governmentality, but also how these may be resisted through material moments of ingestion. As Lavis' exploration of eating disorders in this volume also does, Zivkovik et al. thereby demonstrate that not only do such interventions interfere with, and reposition, bodily materialities, but also that materialities of bodies and foods 'interfere' (Haraway 2008) more profoundly with interventions themselves. This indicates the importance of attending to corporeal and consumable materialities when exploring food and care.

The Bodily Materialities of Careful Eating

Scholars exploring the materiality of food (Bennett 2007, 2010; Carolan 2011; Lavis, forthcoming; Probyn 2000, 2012), argue it to be 'an active inducer-producer of salient, public effects, rather than a passive resource at the disposal of consumers' (Bennett 2007: 45). In turn, Roe shows how 'materiality is displaced during the event of eating, bodies collide, mingle, and separate' (2006: 467). Such scholarship engages with food, thus, as 'more-than-food' (Lorimer 2005. See also Kearnes 2003). In parallel, various ontological developments across the social and physical sciences have recently given rise to a renewed focus on the affective materialities of embodiment as part of this wider turn to materiality (see Blackman 2012; Coole and Frost 2010). This allows a particular approach to corporeality and embodiment as both enfolded in and enacted by encounters between food and care. It emphasizes bodies as at once indeterminate and dynamic, but also as vulnerable to interventions wrapped up as 'care'.

In tandem, but from a differing disciplinary standpoint, critical realist approaches to care have also sought to take account of lived bodily materialities and their wider contexts without resorting to biological reductionism (Williams 1999). Such an engagement casts light on how particular bodies become constructed as in need of care, with wider political discourses coalescing at the level of the individual (Twigg 2006). Yet, it also illuminates the intimacies and tensions involved in caring for an Other's body, highlighting the intrinsic troubling of bodily boundaries in caregiving. Like eating, receiving care through acts such as washing and feeding signify a rupture or re-siting of bodily boundaries in ways potentially pleasurable and painful. To care for an Other's body and to allow another to transgress one's corporeal/territorial boundaries demands both trust and a shifting of power dynamics, as well as questioning of what a body means and where its boundaries lie (see Lawton 2000; Pols 2006, 2013; Twigg 2002). Care may be shared between bodies as multiple bodies become entangled through caring: It is Lindenmeyer's chapter that shows this most explicitly as the clinician-patient relationships she discusses collapse boundaries between those receiving and those giving care. This sense of the coming together of imagined as well as corporeal bodies, as eating and caring is shared between them in ways that trouble easy assumptions of individuality, is also interrogated by Lavis. As such, recognizing the body as entangled in webs of relations produced both by eating and caring, is also to recognize plurality both of and within bodies. It has been suggested that eating is always multiple; it is shared between bodies whilst also making many bodies (Abbots and Lavis 2013; Lavis, forthcoming). Thus, both eating and caring bring into question distinctions between the individual and the multiple. The 'body multiple' (Mol 2002) engendered by both of these acts, and their mobilizations of one another, is one connected to other bodies, human and non-human, and also to practices, technologies, and objects that produce diverse kinds of bodies and ways of being human.

As Twigg concludes, 'focussing on the body also enables us to explore some of the complexities of 'care' as a category of activity' (2006: 173) – one, we suggest that produces and displaces particular bodies. Bodily materialities are not just acted upon, but are also created by discursive formations of food and eating; these, it might be said, 'enable and coordinate the doing of particular kinds of bodies'

(Blackman 2008: 1). It is perhaps a turn to 'viscerality' that has most opened up a way to interrogate relationships between agential bodily materialities and wider biopolitical and cultural structures that are arguably often enfolded in but eclipsed by a focus on caring what Others eat. Viscerality has been defined as 'the sensations, moods and ways of being that emerge from our sensory engagement with the material and discursive environments in which we live' (Longhurst et al. 2009: 334). Developed particularly in the work of Jessica and Allison Hayes-Conroy (e.g. 2010a, 2010b), a turn to viscerality seeks to engage with 'contextualized and interactive versions of the self and other' (2010b: 1273) and establish the centrality of the material body to an exploration of wider political and social structures and interventions. It argues that 'the dynamics of social institutions and/or structures are always already visceral' (ibid.: 1274).

Careful Eating and the Construction of Otherness

Food's power to entangle biological bodies within wider political and cultural structures is a recurrent motif of this volume, and is productively explored across many of the chapters through the lens of otherness. Invoking issues of national identity and belonging, Truninger and Teixera unearth the undercurrent of Portuguese nationalism and 'national taste' in the making of children's bodies in the context of school meals and the education system, whereas Flowers and Swan discuss how multicultural Taste Tours in southwestern Sydney are framed as a means of challenging racism and breaking down ethnic divisions and stereotypes. Flowers and Swan, however, draw attention to the flipside of such initiatives by pointing to the ways in which these can create and reinforce social distance and difference. They thereby indicate how culinary identities and gustatory boundaries are constructed by 'the eating of the Other', and demonstrate how eating can both create and dissolve social and bodily boundaries. Eating is therefore explored in this volume as an intersection through which dynamics between the self and Other are brought into sharp relief (see also Abbots 2013). Food is consequently as much 'a marker of difference' (Caplan 1997: 9) as it is of similarity and while scholarship within Food Studies has accounted for this, it has arguably been less skilled at highlighting the ways that food practices are often as fraught, divisive and tension-filled as they are harmonious and cohesive (Abbots and Lavis 2013; Holtzman 2013; Wilk 2010). This lack is a reflection, perhaps, of a tendency within Food Studies towards, what Holtzman has labelled an ethnography of tasty things (2006) and a Pollyanna-ish inclination for foods that comfort and soothe (2013). As he reminds us, food is 'an arena to create and evoke joys in things that are so close to us but are also a site for tensions, anxieties and regrets' (2013: 145). Comfort can often be discomforting, and closeness claustrophobic.

These wider tensions and ambivalences between proximity and distance, sameness and otherness, and intimacies and estrangements, are all glimpsed in a variety of ways across the chapters of this volume. For example, in Coles' account of chicken consumption in southeast London, place (both imagined and material) is experienced and ingested by middle class professionals who attempt to assuage their food anxieties and insecurities whilst constructing a cosmopolitan identity. The structural class dynamics that Coles explores, both implied and explicit, are just one dimension of how tensions around eating and caring come to the fore, and how the notion of place is employed to construct seemingly caring identities. This thread is also picked up by Abbots, who interrogates how relations of distance are reflected in, and potentially destabilized by, conflicting notions of care-full and care-less foods. Eli et al. also illustrate this multiplicity to care positioning; investigating a web platform, they interrogate how personal care agendas can be made to travel and map across spaces and distances using digital technologies. Social media as a modality of mobilizing care is also taken up in Rousseau's chapter, which demonstrates how counter-discourses of good and proper eating practices are produced through rapid exchanges across cyberspace. Lavis too pays attention to interplays of proximity and distance. By engaging with individuals affected by anorexia, she shows how not eating may enfold wider ethical concerns into self-care by mapping the world in ways both careful and yet painful. In diverse ways, this volume therefore demonstrates that environments and proximities are positioned, and even made, by eating-as-caring for (imagined) places, spaces and Others.

Caring Consumption: Entwining the Personal and Political

The production of Others and selves through careful eating further points to the ways in which the personal and political are entwined in the subjective depths of the body. DuPuis (2000), drawing on David Goodman's (1999) evaluation of actor-network approaches to food, illustrates this process through the lens of organic milk and the 'not-in-my-body' politics of refusal engendered by fears over bovine growth hormone. Challenging perspectives that centre on commodity chains, she stresses the role of the reflexive consumer in the co-production of food systems and interrogates ways in which political activities are played out through everyday food choices. Similarly, Collier and Lakoff (2005) point to the increasing politicization of domestic life and Barnett et al. highlight how 'care, solidarity and collective concern' (2005a: 45) increasingly shape consumer choice and the extent to which ethics are located in domestic lives (Barnett et al. 2005b). This theme of caring consumption is further unpacked in Goodman et al.'s (2011) account of alternative food networks and fair trade which, they point out, are premised on the notion that eating differently can change the world (of food). They demonstrate the role such forms of consumption play in the creation of the moral and ethical self and, in so doing, elucidate how an ethic of care is embedded in fair trade networks. Moreover, for Goodman et al., discourses – or in their words, the 'cultural economies' (ibid.: 209) – of fair trade are more than mere marketing tools: instead they are 'semiotic intermediaries' that are '*indispensable* in creating the meanings of fair trade good as caring consumption' (ibid.: 209-10, emphasis in the original). As such, the 'traffic in things' constitutes the 'traffic in care' (ibid: 209). They thereby not only indicate the relationalities that eating may engender, but also elucidate how these are commoditized, concluding that fair trade 'works to translate the social relations of care into the economic terms of the minimum price and price premium' (ibid. 2016). Care, therefore, can be practised at a distance (Lewis and Potter 2011: 15), albeit through a mechanism that, paradoxically, works to reconnect (Carrier and Leutchford 2012; Kneafsey et al. 2008; Morgan 2010).

Alternative food networks have been subject to further criticism, in part because of their elitist, and often raced and racializing, characteristic (Hayes-Conroy in press; Slocum and Saldhana 2012; West and Domingos 2012). Consequently, questions emerge regarding which social actors have the economic and cultural wherewithal to consume in a 'caring' manner. Or, in other words, following Goodman et al. (2011), who can 'traffic' in care. In this volume, this is considered by Coles as he examines the ways in which middle class sensibilities and anxieties about eating are experienced and enacted by his participants' careful consumption. In so doing, he indicates the class-premised food spaces they inhabit, avoid and imagine. Intersecting with Goodman et al.'s (2011) discussion of fair trade, Coles further highlights the role that the material economy of food, such as labels, plays in making specific networks of production (partially) transparent. He shows how these, often imagined, networks are materially and discursively (re)produced. Weberian notions of class performativity (Weber 1978), and ways in which they intersect with more structural dynamics, are also addressed by Eli et al., Abbots, and Zivkovik et al. These three chapters share an interest in interrogating who has the cultural authority to define the constitution and parameters of careful eating.

The contested production of food knowledges, especially in reference to competing models of 'good' and 'healthy' eating, and the mechanisms through which particular voices are heard and given authority over others, has been subject to some attention (see for example, Abbots and Attala, in press; Flowers and Swan, in press, Rousseau 2012; West et al. 2014). In this volume, Abbots focuses on cultural fairs and examines how notions of tradition interplay with ideas of careful eating, whereas Lavis and Lindenmeyer address clinical contexts. Zivkovic et al. explore the arena of public health, and Truninger and Teixera, the education system. This theme is also key to Eli et al. and Rousseau's explorations of how social media and user-generated content can provide a platform for sharing and challenging information and misinformation about caring foods. But, as Rousseau shows us, new technologies can reinforce and maintain existing cultural hierarchies of knowledge just as much as they can democratize, destablize and give space to new and other voices.

The classed, racialized and gendered dynamics of eating and caring are also seen through the lens of labour relations, specifically in relation to the authority that the performance of reproductive labour both enables and prohibits. The extent to which women continue to perform the majority of food work within the domestic domain has been well established (Counihan and Kaplan 1998;

Pilcher 1998; Weismantel 1988), as has the ways in which women commonly privilege the preferences of family members over their own needs (Counihan 1999; DeVault 1991; Murcott 1983). This 'primary carer' role has been elucidated by Vallianatos and Raine (2008) who argue that the gendered self-definition of the Arabic and South Asian women with whom they researched in Canada rested on their capacity to provision food and cook for their families. Ensuing from such constructions, popular media and public health discourses frequently expound mothers' roles in producing childhood obesity (Maher et al. 2010; Zivkovic et al. 2010). In contrast, Zivkovik et al. show in this volume how such constructions are bound up with affective intimacies in domestic spaces, Flowers and Swan, in turn, demonstrate how such gendered relations of care labour may be enacted outside of the domestic realm as they interrogate the emotional labour of 'hostessing' in the context of culinary tourism. In so doing, their chapter expounds the intersections between gender and ethnicity and the ways in which boundaries of otherness are concomitantly blurred and reinforced through the process of outsourcing and commoditizing care. This theme of outsourcing is further taken up by Truninger and Teixera as they point to the multiple carers involved in the production of Portuguese school meals and, ultimately, children's bodies.

Final Reflections on the Entanglements between Eating and Caring

Elspeth Probyn (2010) reminds us that eating inherently enacts utterly 'messy' concerns. These are concomitantly deliberate and incidental, macro and micro, relational and intimate (Abbots and Lavis 2013: 6). As such, ingesting and digesting involve, and invoke, myriad decisions, actions and consequences through which individuals demonstrate that – and the extent to which – they care about particular issues, people and places. In turn, specific people, places and issues are (ostensibly) cared for through eating and not eating certain foods, places and Others. These complexities, and their multi-dimensionality, shift across and entwine the public and the personal: From consciousness-raising on the public stage and political activism, to everyday moments of shopping and eating, the cultural politics of care are, as the chapters in this volume demonstrate, played out at multiple sites. These include, but are not limited to, individual bodies (Lavis; Zivkovik et al.); kitchens (Truninger and Teixeira); clinical encounters (Lindenmeyer), cultural fairs (Abbots); tourism (Flowers and Swan); the market (Coles) and cyberspace (Eli et al.; Rousseau). Care then, as all of these contributions attest, is a slippery concept that takes on multiple forms and many guises. Although essential to human life and society on the one hand, it may also masquerade, and be wrapped up, as something entirely different from its seemingly intrinsic character. Caring, thus, can appear benign whilst also being politically charged and morally laden; its performances may be as care-less as care-full. Unearthing not only this slippery nature of care, but also how this slipperiness is produced and mobilized draws our attention to the unseemly politics of food more widely. Illustrating how particular bodies, persons and citizens are marginalized and denigrated by carelessly-careful debates around food is a key contribution of this volume, and it is one that intersects with wider concerns regarding food, social justice and the (bio)politics of everyday inequality. As such, asking why and how individuals, groups, institutions and agencies care about what Others eat does not give rise to one simple answer. Rather it engenders a raft of complex responses and reactions that intersect, juxtapose and throw each other into sharp relief. It is those very complexities that we present in this volume and, in so doing, we offer up an intellectual, compassionate, and ultimately humanizing, reflection on what it means to eat, to care and to write about both.

References

Abbots, E-J. 2011. 'It doesn't taste as good from the pet shop': Guinea pig consumption and the performance of class and kinship in Highland Ecuador and New York City. *Food, Culture and Society*, 14(2), 205-24.

Abbots, E-J. 2013. Negotiating foreign bodies: Migration, trust and the risky business of eating in Highland Ecuador, in *Why We Eat, How We Eat: Contemporary Encounters Between Foods and Bodies*, edited by E-J. Abbots and A. Lavis. Farnham: Ashgate, 119-38.

Abbots, E-J. and Attala, L. In press. It's not what you eat but how and that you eat: Social media, counter-discourses and disciplined ingestion among amateur competitive eaters. *Geoforum*.

Abbots, E-J. and Lavis, A. (eds) 2013. *Why We Eat, How We Eat: Contemporary Encounters between Foods and Bodies*. Farnham: Ashgate.

Aphramor, L. Brady, J. and Gingras, J. 2013. Advancing critical dietetics: Theorizing health at every size, in *Why We Eat, How We Eat: Contemporary Encounters between Foods and Bodies*, edited by E-J Abbots and A. Lavis. Farnham: Ashgate, 85-102.

Armstrong, D. 1995. The rise of surveillance medicine. *Sociology of Health and Illness*, 17(3), 393-404.

Baggott, R. 2000. *Public Health: Policy and Politics*. Basingstoke: Palgrave.

Bakhtin, M. 1982. *Dialogic Imagination: Four Essays (New Edition)*. Austin, TX: University of Texas Press.

Barnes, M. 1997. *Care, Communities and Citizens*. Harlow: Addison Wesley Longman.

Barnes, M. 2006. *Caring and Social Justice*. Basingstoke: Palgrave.

Barnes, M. 2012. *Care in Everyday Life: An Ethic of Care in Practice*. Bristol: Policy Press.

Barnett, C., Clarke, N., Cloke, P. and Malpass, A. 2005a. The political ethics of consumerism. *Consumer Policy Review*, 15(2), 45-51.

Barnett, C., Clarke, N., Cloke, P. and Malpass, A. 2005b. Consuming ethics: Articulating the subjects and spaces of ethical consumption. *Antipode*, 37(1), 23-45

Bell, K., McNaughton, D. and Salmon, A. 2009. Medicine, morality and mothering: Public health discourses on foetal alcohol exposure, smoking around children and childhood overnutrition. *Critical Public Health*, 19(2), 155-70.

Bennett, J. 2007. Edible Matter. *New Left Review*, 45 (May-June), 133-45.

Bennett, J. 2010. *Vibrant Matter: A Political Ecology of Things*. Durham, NC: Duke University Press.

Blackman, L. 2008. *The Body: Key Concepts*. Oxford: Berg.

Blackman, L. 2012. *Immaterial Bodies: Affect, Embodiment, Mediation*. London: Sage.

Campbell, J. and Oliver, M. 1996. *Disability Politics: Understanding Our Past, Changing Our Future*. London: Routledge.

Caplan, P. 1997. Approaches to the study of food, health and identity, in *Food, Health and Identity*, edited by P. Caplan. London: Routledge, 1-31.

Carolan, M. 2011. *Embodied Food Politics*. Farnham: Ashgate.

Carrier, J and Leutchford, P. 2012. *Ethical Consumption: Social Value and Economic Practice*. New York and Oxford: Berghahn.

Carsten, J. 1997. *The Heat of the Hearth: The Process of Kinship in a Malay Fishing Community*. Oxford: Clarendon Press.

Collier, S.J. and Lakoff, A. 2005. On regimes of living, in *Global Assemblages: Technology, Politics, and Ethics as Anthropological Problems*, edited by A. Ong and S.J. Collier. Malden: Blackwell.

Colls, R. 2012. Big girls having fun: Reflections on a 'fat accepting space'. *Somatechnics*, 2(1), 18-37.

Connolly, W. 1995. *The Ethos of Pluralisation*. Minneapolis, MN: University of Minnesota Press.

Coole, D. and Frost, S. (eds) 2010. *New Materialisms: Ontology, Agency, and Politics*. Durham, NC: Duke University Press.

Counihan, C.M. 1999. *The Anthropology of Food and the Body: Gender, Meaning and Power*. New York: Routledge.

Counihan, C.M. and Kaplan, S.L. (eds) 1998. *Food and Gender: Identity and Power*. Amsterdam: Harwood.

Crossley, M. L and Crossley, N. 2001. 'Patient' voices, social movements and the habitus: How psychiatric survivors 'speak out'. *Social Science and Medicine*, 52(10), 1477-89.

DeVault, M.L. 1991. *Feeding the Family: The Social Organisation of Caring as Gendered Work*. Chicago, IL: Chicago University Press.

Donini, L., Scardella, P., Piombo, L., Neri, B., Asprino, R. Proietti, A. et al. 2013. Malnutrition in elderly: Social and economic determinants. *The Journal of Nutrition, Health & Aging*, 17(1), 9-15.

DuPuis, E.M. 2000. Not in my body: RBGH and the rise of organic milk. *Agriculture and Human Values*, 17(3), 285-95.

Eli, K. and Lavis, A. 2014. From abject eating to abject being: Representations of obesity in 'Supersize vs. Superskinny', in *Obesity, Eating Disorders, and the Media*, edited by K. Eli and S. Ulijaszek. London: Ashgate, 59-70.

Esplen, E. 2009. *Gender and Care: Overview report* Bridge Development – gender [online]. Available at: http://www.bridge.ids.ac.uk/reports/cep_care_or.pdf [accessed: 15 October 2014].

Faircloth, C. 2010. 'What science says is best': Parenting practices, scientific authority and maternal identity. *Sociological Research Online*, 15(4), np.

Finch, J. and Groves, D. (eds) 1983. *A Labour of Love: Women, Work and Caring*. London: Routledge and Kegan Paul Books.

Fischler, C. 1988. Food, Self and Identity. *Social Science Information*, 27(2), 275-92.

Fisher, B. and Tronto, J. 1990. Toward a feminist theory of caring, in *Circles of Care. Work and Identity in Women's Lives*, edited by E. Abel and M. Nelson. Albany, NY: State University of New York Press, 35-62.

Flowers, R. and Swan, E. In press. *Food Pedagogies*. Farnham: Ashgate.

Foucault, M. 1977. *Discipline and Punish: The Birth of the Prison*. London: Penguin Books.

Foucault, M. 1978. *The History of Sexuality: An Introduction*. New York: Pantheon.

Foucault, M. 1988. Technologies of the Self, in *Technologies of the Self: A Seminar with Michel Foucault*, edited by M. Gutman and P. Hutton. Amherst, MA: The University of Massachusetts Press, 16-49.

Foucault, M. 2003. *The Birth of the Clinic: An Archaeology of Medical Perception*. London and New York: Routledge Classics.

Gilligan, C. 1982. *In a Different Voice: Psychological Theory and Women's Development*. Cambridge, MA: Harvard University Press.

Goodman, D. 1999. Agro-food studies in the 'age of ecology': Nature, corporeality, bio-politics. *Sociologia Ruralis*, 39(1), 17-38.

Goodman, D., DuPuis, E.M. and Goodman, M.K. 2011. *Alternative Food Networks: Knowledge, Practice and Politics*. Oxford: Routledge.

Guthman, J. 2011. *Weighing In: Obesity, Food Justice, and the Limits of Capitalism*. Berkeley, CA and Los Angeles, CA: University of California Press.

Haraway, D. 2008. Otherwordly conversations, terran topics, local terms, in *Material Feminisms*, edited by S. Alaimo and S. Hekman. Bloomington, IN: Indiana University Press, 157-87

Hayes-Conroy, J. In press. *Savoring Alternative Food: School Gardens, Healthy Eating and Visceral Difference*. Abingdon: Routledge.

Hayes-Conroy, A. and Hayes-Conroy, J. 2010a. Visceral difference: Variations in feeling (slow) food. *Environment and Planning*, A 42, 2956-71.

Hayes-Conroy, J. and Hayes-Conroy, A. 2010b. Visceral geographies: Mattering, relating and defying. *Geography Compass*, 4(9), 1273-82.

Held, V. 2006. *The Ethics of Care: Personal, Political and Global*. Oxford: Oxford University Press.

Hinchliffe, S. 2007. *Geographies of Nature: Societies, Environments, Ecologies* London: Sage.

Holtzman, J.D. 2006. Food and memory. *Annual Review of Anthropology*, 35(1), 361-78.

Holtzman, J. 2013. Reflections on fraught food, in *Why We Eat, How We Eat: Contemporary Encounters Between Foods and Bodies*, edited by E-J. Abbots and A. Lavis. Farnham: Ashgate, 139-46.

Inthorn, S. and Boyce, T. 2010. 'It's disgusting how much salt you eat!' Television discourses of obesity, health and morality. *International Journal of Cultural Studies*, 13(1), 83-100.

Kearnes M. 2003. Geographies that matter: The rhetorical deployment of physicality? *Social and Cultural Geography*, 4(2), 139-52.

Klein, J. and Murcott, A. (eds) 2014. *Food Consumption in Global Perspective: Essays in the Anthropology of Food in Honour of Jack Goody.* Basingstoke: Palgrave Macmillan.

Kneafsey, M. Cox, R. Holloway, L. Dowler, E. Venn, L. and Tuomainen, H. 2008. *Reconnecting Consumers, Producers and Food: Exploring Alternatives.* Oxford: Berg.

Kubiak, C., Rogers, A. and Turner, A. 2007. *A Path of Crazy Paving: Tension in Workbased Learning in Health and Social Care.* Milton Keynes: Open University.

Lavin, C. 2013. *Eating Anxieties.* Minneapolis, MN: University of Minnesota Press.

Lavis, A. 2014. Engrossing encounters: Materialities and metaphors of fat in the lived experiences of individuals with anorexia, in *Fat: Culture and Materiality*, edited by C. Forth and A Leitch. London: Bloomsbury, 91-108.

Lavis, A. forthcoming. Imagined materialities and material imaginings: Foods, bodies and the 'stuff' of (not) eating. *Gastronomica.*

Lawton, J. 2000. *The Dying Process: Patients' Experiences of Palliative Care.* London: Routledge.

Lewis, G., Gewirtz, S. and Clarke, J. (eds) 2000. *Rethinking Social Policy.* London: Sage.

Lewis, T and A. Potter. (eds) 2011. *Ethical Consumption: A Critical Introduction.* London: Routledge.

Longhurst, R., Johnston, L. and Ho, E. 2009. A visceral approach: Cooking 'at home' with migrant women in Hamilton, New Zealand. *Transactions of the Institute of British Geographers*, 34(3), 333-45.

Lorimer, H. 2005. Cultural Geography: The busyness of being 'more-than-representational'. *Progress in Human Geography*, 29(1), 83-94.

Lupton, D. 1996. *Food, the Body and the Self.* London, Thousand Oaks and New Delhi: Sage.

Lupton, D. 1997. Foucault and the medicalisation critique, in *Foucault, Health and Medicine*, edited by A. Petersen and R. Bunton. London and New York: Routledge, 94-110.

Maher, J., Fraser, S. and Wright, J. 2010. Framing the mother: Childhood obesity, maternal responsibility and care. *Journal of Gender Studies*, 19(3), 233-47.

Mills, M. 1992. *The Politics of Dietary Change.* Aldershot: Dartmouth.

Mol A. 2002. *The Body Multiple: Ontology in Medical Practice.* Durham, NC and London: Duke University Press.

Mol, A. 2008. *The Logic of Care: Health and the Problem of Patient Choice.* London: Routledge.

Mol, A., Moser, I. and Pols, J. (eds) 2010a. *Care in Practice: On Tinkering in Clinics, Homes and Farms.* New London: Transaction Publishers.

Mol, A, Moser, I. and Pols, J. 2010b. Care: Putting practice into theory, in *Care in Practice: On Tinkering in Clinics, Homes and Farms*, edited by A. Mol et al. New London: Transaction Publishers, 7-26.

Morgan, K. 2010. Local and green, global and fair: The ethical foodscape and the politics of care. *Environment and planning.* A 42 1852-67.

Murcott, A. 1983 'It's a pleasure to cook for him': Food, mealtimes and gender in some south Wales households, in *The Public and the Private: Social Patterns of Gender Relations*, edited by E. Garmanikow, D. Morgan, J. Purvis and D. Taylorson. London: Heinemann, 78-90.

Murray, S. 2005. (Un/be)coming out? Rethinking fat politics. *Social Semiotics*, 15(2), 153-63.

Oullette, L. and Hay, J. 2008. Makeover television, governmentality and the good citizen. *Continuum: Journal of Media & Cultural Studies*, 22(4), 471-84.

Petersen A. and Lupton D. (eds) 1996. *The New Public Health. Health and Self in the Age of Risk.* London: Sage.

Pierson, C.A. 1999. Ethnomethodological analysis of account of feeding demented residents in long-term care. *Journal of Nursing Scholarship*, 31(2), 127-31.

Pilcher, J.M. 1998. *Que Vivan Los Tamales! Food and the Making of Mexican Identity.* Albuquerque: University of New Mexico Press.

Pols, J. 2006. Accounting and washing – Good care in long-term psychiatry. *Science, Technology, & Human Values*, 31(4), 409-30.

Pols, J. 2013. Washing the patient: Dignity and aesthetic values in nursing care. *Nursing Philosophy*, 14(3), 186-200.

Probyn, E. 2000. *Carnal Appetites: Food, Sex, Identities*. London: Routledge.

Probyn, E. 2010. Feeding the world: Towards a messy ethics of eating, in *A Critical Introduction to Consumption*, edited by E. Potter and T. Lewis. London: Routledge, 103-15.

Probyn, E. 2012. Eating roo: Of things that become food. *New Formations*, 74(1), 33-45.

Qureshi, H. and Walker, A. 1989. *The Caring Relationship: Elderly People and their Families.* Basingstoke: Macmillan Educational.

Ray, K. 2004. *The Migrant's Table: Meals and Memories in Bengali-American Households*. Philadelphia, PA: University of Pennsylvania Press.

Renne, E.P. 2007. Mass producing food traditions for West Africans abroad. *American Anthropologist*, 109(4), 616-25.

Roe, E. 2006. Material connectivity, the immaterial and the aesthetic of eating practices: An argument for how genetically modified foodstuff becomes inedible. *Environment and Planning A*, 38, 465-81.

Rousseau, S. 2012. *Food Media: Celebrity Chefs and the Politics of Everyday Interference*. London: Berg.

Saber, G. and Posner, R. 2013. Remembering the past and constructing the future over a communal plate. *Food, Culture and Society*, 16(2), 197-222.

Slocum, R. and Saldanha, A. (eds) 2013. *Geographies of Race and Food: Fields, Bodies, Markets*. Farnham: Ashgate.

Stearns, C. 1999. Breastfeeding and the good maternal body. *Gender & Society*, 13(3), 308-25.

Stewart, K. 2007. *Ordinary Affects*. Durham, NC: Duke University Press.

Thomas, C. 1993. Deconstructing concepts of care. *Sociology*, 27(4), 646-69.

Tronto, J. 1993. *Moral Boundaries: A Political Argument for an Ethic of Care*. London: Routledge.

Trussell Trust. 2014. 'The Trussell Trust's UK foodbank network' [online]. Available at: http://www.trusselltrust.org/resources/documents/Press/TT-Foodbank-Information-Pack-2013-14.pdf [accessed: 3 October 2014].

Tuomainen, H.M. 2009. Ethnic identity, (post)colonialism and foodways: Ghanaians in London. *Food, Culture and Society*, 12(4), 525-54.

Twigg, J. 2002. *Bathing: The Body and Community Care*. London: Routledge.

Twigg, J. 2006. *The Body in Health and Social Care*. Basingstoke: Palgrave Macmillan.

Twigg, J. and Atkin, K. 1994. *Carers Perceived: Policy and Practice in Informal Care*. Milton Keynes: Open University Press.

Ungerson, C. 1983. Why do women care?, in *A Labour of Love: Women, Work and Caring*, edited by J. Finch and D. Groves. London: Routledge and Kegan Paul Books, 41-9.

Ungerson, C. 2005. Care, work and feeling. *The Sociological Review*, 53(2), 188-203.

Vallianatos, H. and K. Raine. 2008. Consuming food and constructing identities among Arabic and south Asian immigrant women. *Food, Culture and Society*, 11(3), 355-73.

Walkerdine, V. 2003. Reclassifying upward mobility: Femininity and the neo-liberal subject. *Gender and Education*, 15(3), 237-48.

Weber, M. 1978. *Economy and Society: An Outline of Interpretative Sociology (Volumes 1 & 2)*, edited by G. Roth and C. Wittich. Berkeley, CA: University of California Press.

Weismantel, M. 1988. *Food, Gender and Poverty in the Ecuadorian Andes* Philadelphia, PA: University of Pennsylvania Press.

West, H.G and Domingos, N. 2012. Gourmandizing poverty food: The Serpa cheese slow food presidium. *Journal of Agrarian Change*, 12(1), 120-43

West, H, Domingos, N. and Sobral, J. (eds) 2014. *Food Between the Country and the City: Changing Ethnographies of a Global Foodscape*. London: Bloomsbury.

WHO 2000. *Obesity: Preventing and Managing the Global Epidemic*. WHO Technical Report Series 894. Geneva: World Health Organisation.

Wilk, R. 2010. Power at the table. Food fights and happy meals. *Cultural Studies: Critical Methodologies*, 10(6), 428-36.

Williams, S.J. 1999. Is anybody there? Critical realism, chronic illness and the disability debate. *Sociology of Health and Illness*, 21(6), 797-819.

Wright, J. and Harwood, V. 2009. *Biopolitics and the 'Obesity Epidemic': Governing Bodies*. New York: Routledge.

Zivkovic, T., Warin, M., Davies, M. and Moore, V. 2010. In the name of the child: The gendered politics of childhood obesity. *Journal of Sociology*, 46(4), 375-92.

PART I
Eating to Care: Proximities and Productions

This opening part explores ways in which the act of eating produces, mobilizes and ruptures dynamics of care. Extending explorations of how individuals care for themselves and Others through their food choices, this part begins the volume's narrative arc by asking what relationships, discourses and imaginings of care are embedded not only in individuals' eating practices, but also in the ways they articulate their food preferences *vis-à-vis* other individuals and social groups. These processes are examined through the diverse contexts of culinary tours, social media debates, and celebrations of traditional food. As such, the central argument that care is a slippery concept that takes multiple forms and guises – and that this slipperiness enables caring to be politically deployed – starts to emerge. The chapters in this part all demonstrate that eating is an act inherently productive of, as well as entangled in, social relations – whether these are between ethnic groups, social classes or just individuals with conflicting views on what comprises 'good' food. All elucidate how these relations dynamically take shape through everyday engagement and proximity with Others. In so doing, each points to the ways that eating, eating the Other, and caring about the eating of Others demonstrate and enact relationships of care. In turn, careless eating – that is not eating in preferred manners and adopting foods considered less desirable – is shown to be constructed as a problematic practice that requires intervention and interference in the forms of, for example, health fairs, education and the instigation of online debates. Collectively, then, this part draws attention to the ways in which individuals ingesting careful foods are constituted as more caring than those who do not. In short, to eat (certain foods) is to care (for and about particular people and issues).

By tracing the often fraught and tension-filled nature of these processes, the chapters in this part further examine ways that subjective knowledges of proper eating are overlaid onto particular individuals or segments of society including, for example, ethnic women in the form of hostesses or members of the peasantry. They thereby indicate how particular social groups are expected to eat carefully, and the ways in which this intersects with ethnicity, gender, class, and body size. They further examine how these expectations are both upheld and challenged through social interactions. This part consequently highlights the political dynamics of care, the (moral) authority of the carer, and the eater as carer.

Chapter 1

Multiculturalism as Work: The Emotional Labour of Ethnic Food Tour Guides

Rick Flowers and Elaine Swan

Introduction

In this chapter, we examine the complex gendered and racialized politics of caring work performed by guides on Taste Tours, a food-tourism social enterprise. The tours are organized by The Benevolent Society, Australia's oldest not-for-profit organization and run in southwestern Sydney. They are 'designed to show the very best of southwest Sydney's amazing multicultural food traditions' as a means 'to bridge cultural divides and build community pride, generate income for local businesses, and create training and employment opportunities' (The Benevolent Society 2011). Southwestern Sydney has a large migrant population and has long been represented in racist ways in the media and public imaginary (Poynting et al. 2004; White 2004). The tours are presented as attempts at countering such 'negative perceptions', thus creating a more 'caring' and 'careful' image of the region and its people through food.

A diverse organization with approximately 850 staff and 600 volunteers, The Benevolent Society provides a range of services focused on children, older people and women's health (Michaux 2010). It was established in 1813, only 30 years after the British First Fleet invaded Australia, to 'promote missionary work and the 'sacred duties of religion' (Clarke 2013: np). Originally called the NSW Society for Promoting Christian Knowledge and Benevolence, in 1818 it was renamed The Benevolent Society of NSW, and became a non-religious organization with the remit of providing 'relief of the poor, the distressed, the aged, and the infirm, and for other benevolent purposes' (ibid.: np). Since that time the society has extended its service provision to maternity services, home care, child protection, community development and more recently social enterprise activity. It derives most of its funding from government grants, and donors and recently income from social enterprises.

Against this backdrop, Taste Tours has been running for three years as a social enterprise. In essence, this means that the tours are organized as a business with a social purpose. Fee-income is reinvested back into the business and the community. Although somewhat contested, social enterprises are often imagined as more 'caring' organizational forms than those which are for-profit (Haugh

2005: 5). Taste Tours is described as 'designed to give something back to the local community' (The Benevolent Society 2011).

Failed Multiculturalism

In order to understand the aims of Taste Tours, it is important to know that there has been a longstanding economic and cultural marginalization of southwestern Sydney (Poynting et al. 2004). It has large numbers of migrants and refugees from southern and eastern Europe, Vietnam, the Middle East and Africa; is relatively poor; and is the target of racist and Islamaphobic media and political constructions about 'ethnic' violent crime, the 'criminalized Arab,' and ethnic young men's 'gangs', such that some major suburbs are portrayed as 'no-go' enclaves for Anglo-Celtic Australians (Collins 2009; Dreher 2003; Noble 2009). As a result, there has been a repeated demonization of categories such as the 'Arab', 'Muslim', 'Middle Eastern' and 'Lebanese' in the reporting of events in the region and racial discrimination and violence towards men and women from these backgrounds. Because of this context of 'Othering' Vietnamese, Arab and Muslim Australians, southwestern Sydney is constructed as Australian multiculturalism 'gone wrong' (Dreher 2003). It is these negative 'Othering' perceptions of crime and danger, and the effects of these on small ethnic businesses, that Taste Tours seeks to 'rewrite' through ethnic neighbourhood tourism and the work of the guides.

Eating the Other

Ethnic culinary tourism is one of a number of concerted efforts to construct 'ethnic' food as a medium through which people learn about other cultures and as a sign that they, their cities and regions are more 'tolerant' of difference, more caring of the Other (Duruz 2010; Flowers and Swan 2012, 2015; Hage 1997; Probyn 2000; Sheridan 2000). Thus in Australia, ethnic food has 'long been the acceptable face of multiculturalism' (Gunew 1993: 41). There has been much debate on the ethics, politics and effects of such culinary tourism. The term 'eating the Other', taken from bell hooks' (1992) critique of the commodification and consumption of racial difference by white people, has been taken up in food studies to characterize the way that white middle-class people consume ethnic food as a form of cultural capital production. For hooks, dominant white cultures visually or metaphorically eat racialized bodies to spice up the blandness of mainstream white culture (Sheller 2003). Through commodification, the Other's histories of racism and imperialism are decontextualized in a process of 'commodity fetishism' (hooks 1992). Hence, writers suggest that white people learn an attenuated idea of Others' cultures and the historical, political, colonial contexts of their lives and foods (Hage 1997; Heldke 2003; hooks 1992).

At the centre of the critique is the idea that the Other is simply used as an object for a white project of narcissist self-development and status enhancement: one might say the consumer is careless and self-centred through their food. For writers such as Ghassan Hage (1997) and Lisa Heldke (2003), the greed of the eater for parading their cultural competence gets in the way of any care for the workers in ethnic restaurants, or the socio-cultural histories of their food and journeys as migrants or refugees. For Hage, it is a detached intellectual project lacking any sensory relationship to the materiality of food or actual engagement with local people (1997: 86). Eating the Other is thus a form of self-care, learning more about the self, with the desire to be oneself by getting closer to and incorporating the stranger. Eating the Other is more about appetite than generosity, and narcissism than altruism (Ahmed 2002).

A question arising from this debate is whether the Other can be eaten in a more caring and careful way. In one school of thought, Heldke sets out an anti-colonial project of eating the Other in which careful eating entails 'self-reflective eating' (2003: 117), learning how colonialism structures experiences of eating ethnic food and developing a more ongoing relationship with ethnic food producers – a more attentive sociality. In another school of thought, careful eating of the Other happens through 'everyday multiculturalism' (Wise and Velayutham 2009: 1): the ways multi-ethnic people have prosaic encounters and ongoing interactions in neighbourhood and everyday settings such as schools, buses, shops, community gardens, and sports fields. These interactions, so the argument goes, produce a more caring relation to the Other than a version of multiculturalism which relies on celebrations and festivals (Jakubowicz and Ho 2014; Wise 2010; Wise and Velayutham 2009). A third school of thought suggests that the sensory and embodied aspects of ethnic food encounters produce a visceral connection to the Other in positive ways (Highmore 2008; Johnston and Longhurst 2012; Molz 2007). In this view, eating the Other in tourist encounters displays a physical as well as an intellectual stance of openness toward consuming difference, with tourists voluntarily seeking out a sense of risk and curiosity through ethnic food, and alienation which can result from eating unfamiliar food (Molz 2007: 82-5). These produce what Amanda Wise calls 'hopeful intercultural encounters' producing new ways of thinking and doing (2005: 172. See also Johnston and Longhurst 2012).

For Hage (1997) and Uma Narayan (1997), the focus needs to be on the agency of the Other in producing food-multiculturalism. Thus, Hage writes of the ethical importance of researching the Other as subject: what he calls the 'feeder, not just the white cosmopolitan 'eater'. With these ideas in mind, in this chapter, we examine the caring work of the migrant women guides on Taste Tours. Over a 12-month period in 2012 and 2013 we undertook participant observation research on five tours, conducted a focus-group interview with five guides, plus one-on-one interviews. We participated in the tours, walking, eating, drinking and conversing with the guides, tourists and shopkeepers, undertaking what has been called 'tourist-ethnography' (Jack and Phipps 2005). We audio-taped and transcribed the focus groups and interviews. From this participant observation we produced data in the form of photographs and fieldnotes. Using a loosely grounded theory (Charmaz 2014) approach, we followed a coding process augmented by memo-writing. We drew on literature on guiding work and emotional labour for our analysis and from the outset we were clear that we would use etic categories informed by critical race and feminist theories and thus positioning us closer to 'critical' ethnography than traditional ethnography.

Taste Tours: Ethnic Neighbourhood and Benevolent Tourism

The Taste Tours program began in 2010 with a half-day walking tour in the suburb of Bankstown. It continues to expand with tours now being offered in seven other suburbs of southwestern Sydney. Names of tours include Babylonian Delights, South American Food Trail, Shanghai to Saigon, and World Explorer and typically participants to these tours will get to shop for and taste foods originating from various language groups and countries in the Middle East, Southeast Asia and South America. It should be noted that they are all multi-ethnic food tours.

Their website describes the tours as follows:

> All tours are led by local guides and hosted by businesses that share their stories of food and culture. We reveal the best places to eat and shop, all while you enjoy a feast for the senses. You'll also get a sample bag to fill to bursting point with goodies collected along the way. *Taste* is far from your typical food tour. Let local guides share their secrets on the best places to eat and shop for authentic dishes and ingredients.

There are usually between ten and 20 tourists on a tour and the guides work in pairs, with one leading the group and the other bringing up the rear, wheeling a trolley of samples, information and serviettes. Typically, a tour includes visits to three or four shops, one café and one restaurant, with time at each stop for a talk by the guides, shopping and sampling of foods.

In 2012, at the time of our fieldwork, the guides were all women, residents of southwestern Sydney and from non-Anglo Australian ethnic backgrounds: Lebanese, Chinese, Greek, Maltese, Egyptian and Pakistani. Guides were aged between 30 and 50 and most were second-generation, but some recently-arrived, migrants. They are not employees of The Benevolent Society but contracted on a freelance basis. As the literature on guiding work suggests, the work of the guides is highly varied (Bunten 2008; Cohen 1985; Salazar 2008; Valtonen 2009). And we observed that the Taste Tours guides are highly skilled, drawing on various kinds of expertise. Broadly speaking, they provide tourists with formal information about the suburb, and the businesses being visited; factual plus entertaining information about foods, and culture; marshal the group from its meeting point to the variety of shops, cafés and restaurants on the tour; answer individual and group queries on a range of topics; keep the group on time to the agenda; build group conviviality; and liaise with each business.

On the programme's website at the time of our research, the ethnic women were positioned as housewives and mothers who cook for love. In fact, most Taste Tours guides have university qualifications and some demonstrate considerable professional pride not only in their knowledge of multi-ethnic foods but also ability to lead and facilitate a group of tourists. By positioning them less as professionals and more as local residents, The Benevolent Society may be creating a sense of 'authenticity' for tourists but are devaluing the work of the guides. We elaborate on this in the rest of this chapter by analysing the emotional labour the guides invest in performing their role.

Taste Tours can be understood as a form of 'ethnic neighbourhood tourism' (Santos et al. 2008). While this type of tourist activity is small-scale, in cities that are 'culturally diverse', there is a growing trend to make local neighbourhoods destinations for 'tourists' from within the same city. Such tours capitalize on the 'ethnic' products of neighbourhoods by 'offering entertaining representations of their culture and history and drawing attention to charged relations between ethnicity and the ... urban landscape' (Santos et al. 2008: 1002). Touristification of previously marginalized ethnic neighbourhoods is seen to bring benefits including economic development, 'cultural revitalization' and cross-cultural understanding. There are, however, concerns in the emergent literature about whose version of culture is produced in the 'touristification' of ethnic neighbourhoods' and how this can amplify rather than counter racial stereotypes circulating in the media (Conforti 1996; Santos et al. 2008).

The caring work of the guides is not only shaped by a wider cultural discourse of eating the Other and ethnic neighbourhood tourism, it is inflected by the history and policies of The Benevolent Society and connotations of benevolence. Taste Tours is described on their website as 'eating for a good cause'. This refers to the aims of enabling intercultural learning, community pride, job creation and economic development. Interestingly in relation to this, the concept of benevolence in Christian tradition is defined as:

> An attitude of the mind and heart that wishes the best for one's neighbour ...
> benevolence is both comprehensive and universal. It wishes all good things for
> the neighbour and it recognises the neighbour as everyone – including one's
> enemies. (Glaser 1994: 111)

But there is, of course, a politics of benevolence where 'doing good' is vigorously contested and particularly so in relation to race and power. Damien Riggs (2004) argues that in political circles, 'white benevolence' in Australia has been constructed as a challenge to Indigenous sovereignty. In essence, the concept of benevolence says our intentions are good; look at the good things we do, rather than showing how white people benefit from race privilege and the legacy of colonialism.

We are presenting a framework to analyse the caring work of tour guides that draws links between the politics of benevolence, ethnic neighbourhood tourism and eating the Other. A strategy to make links between these bodies of literature is to analyse the ways tourist expectations are formed. Tourist expectations are the ideas and imaginaries about destinations with which tourists arrive and these, in turn, shape how guides behave (Salazar 2010; Skinner and Theodossopoulos 2011). Thus, tourists have individual 'pre-tour understandings' (Bruner 2010, cited in Salazar ibid.: xiii) informed by widely-circulating political and cultural stereotypes and discourses (Salazar 2010). These 'travel' through documentaries, art, museums, photographs, postcards, travelogues, blogs, websites, guidebooks and brochures, news coverage, academic publications, literature, advertising and television (ibid.: 9). Ideas about ethnic neighbourhood tours can be affected by historical forms of 'othering' and racism together with discourses of celebratory urban multiculturalism (Santos et al. 2008).

Tourism websites form part of this circulation. Taste Tours has had lots of coverage in national and local newspapers, positioning them within food multiculturalism and social enterprise discourses. To get to the Taste Tours webpages, potential tourists have to go through The Benevolent Society's main website. This is where potential tourists find information about the tours and the guides, and make bookings. The Benevolent Society's website frames the caring agenda in relation to Taste Tours in particular ways. It is positioned in relation to the Benevolent Society's history of 'doing' benevolence.

Caring Work and Emotional Labour

Drawing on critical race theories and feminist research on emotional labour and hostessing in the context of tourism we present an analysis of guides' work – practices of care – against a backdrop of racism, Islamophobia and fear. It is against this backdrop that we make connections between a politics of eating the Other and emotional labour. The guides' emotional labour is racialized and gendered in multiple ways.

As a form of tourism-work, guiding is complex, multifaceted and intricate. It encompasses a range of intellectual, manual, educational, emotional and social skills (Bunten 2008; Valtonen 2009), as we learned first-hand from observing and talking to the *Taste Tour* guides. Soile Veijola (2009a) argues that it is the 'service-work' aspect as opposed to these other elements of tour guiding which is now most significant for tourism. Hence guides are expected to be friendly, amiable and sociable, take care of the group's needs, keep the group in a good mood, manage tensions, relax the group and create a comforting social atmosphere (Veijola 2009a. See also Wong and Wang 2009: 250). We examine this relational work through the concept of emotional labour, defined by Arlie Hoschchild as 'the emotional style of offering the service as part of the service itself (1983: 16, cited in Veijola and Valtonen 2007: 16). For example, Mike Crang (1997) describes how tourism workers are required to express emotional work such as deference, eagerness to please, and friendliness and to produce affective customer experiences in the here and now of the social situation.

Relational caring service-work is theorized as a further extension of the cultural feminization of labour. This is because it draws on emotional, aesthetic, domestic and social skills of femininity (Adkins 2005; Gray 2003; Lovell 2000; Swan 2008; Veijola 2009b). Women perform most of this service work, although increasingly it is also expected from male workers. In this line of argument, Veijola and Jokinen (2008) suggest that the best way to characterize the provision of care in tourism is through the concept of 'hostessing'. By this, they mean the work of attending to the emotional, bodily and social needs of tourists which requires the core skills of a good hostess or housewife – the capacity to relate, take care and host. They write: 'femininity is foundational to the acts and images of hospitality and care-taking' (ibid.: 42).

In this view, caring service-work in guiding is emotional labour and tour guides are expected to 'express positive emotions and to supress negative ones' (Wong and Wang 2008: 252). For example, guides need to produce amiableness, considerateness, friendliness and warmth in themselves; and relaxation, satisfaction and openness in tourists. As Veijola argues it is about 'the importance of smiling and showing *a will to please* (2009b: 16). Hostessing then involves the whole spectrum of bodily feeling, intellectual and communicative capacities and expertise encompassing the body, voice, intonation, facial gestures. But emotional labour is constrained by the cultural means for 'pleasing' such as size, looks, attire, attitude, age and gender (ibid.: 21). For Veijola subservience is at its centre.

Hostessing is about the gendering of the work itself and the separation of gender from the worker. There are two points worth noting here. First, claims to performances of femininity as workplace resources are not evenly distributed or rewarded (Adkins 2005). Not everyone can mobilize their gender at will (Skeggs 2004: 53). This is because hostessing skills are not seen as expertise or skill but as 'as part of their nature to please others and not their professional know-how' (Jokinen and Veijola 2012: 39. See also Bolton 2009). Thus, the terms under which women and men perform hostessing and claim workplace rewards and consequences are unequal (Adkins 2005; Swan 2008; Veijola and Jokinen 2008).

Secondly, there is an emotional burden of a work-culture where 'the discipline of "customer is always right" is pervasive in service settings' (Wong and Wang 2008: 251). Thus, a mobilization of gender performance does not count unless it is recognized as having audience effects (Adkins 2005: 123, cited in Veijola 2009b). In other words, employee effectiveness is not measured on the basis of product quality but on terms related to customers; workers therefore focus attention on the effects of their labour on the intended audience (Adkins 2005: 122-3, cited in Veijola 2009b). This means caring is reproduced under unequal and sometimes coercive power relations in which 'the customer is always right' (e.g. Veijola and Valtonen 2007). The audience act as the 'final judge' (ibid.: 20). This is further exacerbated by the plethora of customer surveys, ratings, and job descriptions that 'foreground customer care, comfort, pleasure and contentment' (Adkins 2005: 122. See also Veijola and

Valtonen 2007). This results in a 'tight feedback loop' between self-surveillance of emotions and intended audience effects (Veijola 2009: 120).

In their work on tour guides, Jehn-Yih Wong and Chih-Hung Wang suggest that when guides are expected to lead tourists in ways that make them satisfied and happy, it is sometimes at the expense of what the guides may believe and feel. This adds an extra challenge for the emotional labour of tour guides because they have so little time off-stage in 'which to release the emotional burden' (2009: 250). As has been noted, 'privileged' emotion managers have more autonomy and freedom in relation to their emotional expression and are provided with more organisational resources – time, space, buffers and training – to enable them to manage their feelings and produce an emotional performance (MacDonald and Sirianni 1996). In turn, this exacerbates the existing inequalities in the emotional exchange between tourists and guides (Bolton and Houlihan 2005).

Veijola and Valtonen note that occupational racism means that caring work is imagined to 'suit' migrants, but they still do not consider emotional labour in racialized terms. In fact, generally little attention has been given to the racialization of emotion-work (Mirchandani 2003, 2012). Thus, much of the scholarship relies on a falsely universalist conceptualization of emotion and gender (Gunarathnam and Lewis 2001; Mirchandani 2003, 2012). In essence, the literature on emotional labour has ignored the differential affectivity of racially minoritized men and women (Ahmed 2012; Ramos-Zayas 2012; Tolia-Kelly 2009).

The racialization of emotional labour can be understood in a number of ways. First, there are distinct 'feeling-rules' for racialized minorities in workplaces, inflected by class and gender (Froyum 2013; Ramos-Zayas 2012; Shan 2012; Wingfield 2010). These shape expectations about what racialized minorities are expected to feel, how they express what they feel and how their feelings are interpreted (Froyum 2013; Wingfield 2010). Secondly, emotional labour results from and is part and parcel of racial inequality. Research shows how racialized men and women are expected to suppress criticism of inequality and racism, to show 'extraordinary emotional restraint' (Wilkins 2012: 35. See also Froyum 2013; Michandani 2003). Thirdly, social theorists have emphasized the importance of understanding the cultural racialization of emotion and care historically (Anderson 2000; Glenn 1992; Spelman 2008); for example, Elizabeth Spelman (2008) has argued that black people in America have been expected to labour at caring for whiteness. Emotional labour, then, is not universal but highly stratified and differentiated racially and by class.

Emotional labour then needs to be understood as racialized in its 'form, content and consequences' (Froyum 2013: 1071), which has implications for guiding and tourism service work. As Ana Ramos-Zayas (2012) writes, emotional labour based on being 'friendly' is critical to the formation of the neoliberal personhood. But this style requires access to resources and audience reception for its successful performance. These may be unevenly distributed and with the ability to be friendly and to be seen as friendly by others, profoundly classed, racialized and gendered (Tolia-Kelly 2009). Audience reception of emotions is racialized as Sara Ahmed

(2004a) shows: feelings such as fear stick to some bodies and not others. Not everyone has the right bodily techniques for emotional labour norms, nor can they turn their emotions into workplace resources.

Critical race theorists challenge the idea prevalent in much of the emotional labour literature that feelings are something we possess internally and then express. Rather 'emotions produce the effect of surfaces and boundaries of bodies' (Ahmed 2012: 10). Hence, Ahmed writes of feelings as impressions: impressions we have of others and impressions we make on others (2012: 47). But emotions do not circulate between us smoothly or freely as some bodies remind us of histories that are disturbing (Ahmed 2012: 54). Racism then is a particular:

> form of contact between others … it is not simply that the subject feels hate, or feels fear, nor is it the case that the subject is simply hateful or is fearsome: the emotions of hate and fear are shaped by the 'contact zone' in which others impress upon us, and as well as leave their impressions. (Ahmed 2012: 194)

Past histories of contact mean that a racial Other can be perceived as threatening, fearful or disgusting. 'These histories have already impressed upon the surface of the bodies at the same time as they create new impressions' (Ahmed 2012: 194). In this way, emotions work performatively: in reading the Other as threatening, or disgusting, we become filled up with fear or disgust.

Extending Ahmed's conceptualization of emotions, Michele Lobo (2014) argues that whiteness in Australia works as a force that exerts affective pressures on racialized bodies in public spaces. These pressures have the 'potential to wound, numb and immobilise bodies affecting what they can do or what they can become' (Lobo 2014: 1). Whiteness materializes through 'racialized mis-interpellation and bodily intensities of hurt, anger and frustration' (ibid.: 2). Racism thus 'sucks out life' fragmenting and shattering (Hage 2008, cited in Lobo 2014: 104). To counter such shattering intensities requires the mobilization of affect by racially minoritized Others to capacitate bodies to inhabit public spaces.

In summary, emotional labour understood as hostessing is a productive way to analyse an important element of the work of the tour guides on Taste Tours. But, as often conceived, it does not get at how emotional labour is racialized. The scholarship by critical race theorists asks us to reflect on how hostessing skills and expertise may be differentially and unequally produced and received, and require more labour in response to racism, its impressions and forces by racially minoritized tourist workers such as the tour guides.

Caring Work on Taste Tours

> As a guide you have to notice the overall tone of the tour and see what's needed. So you can actually tell when people are losing interest … You have to stop and then change the tone and lift things up. So there's a general feeling that you

get. It's like an over-riding tone in your head at all times, monitoring that in the background.

This first quotation comes from a guide regularly employed by Taste Tours who is an Australian woman of Maltese heritage. We start here as this quote exemplifies how she and other guides see the intensity of keeping tourists happy as a critical part of the work they do. Caring work for the guides also entails researching and presenting information about the extensive range of 'ethnic' food ingredients, the tourist-site history and building relationships with local shopkeepers, although we noted that this form of labour was less discussed by the guides. Rather, the guides placed emphasis on their emotional labour and relational caring work such as monitoring and transforming the emotional climate of the group. This work also involves producing a group from a rag-tag of individuals (Valtonen 2009).

Emotional labour has to start at the very beginning of the tour when the guides create a welcoming friendly atmosphere and start to cohere the group. The following excerpt from our fieldnotes describes the work of two guides at the beginning of a multi-ethnic tour in Bankstown in southwestern Sydney:

> The guides start by welcoming people at the railway station. The lead-guide is a Lebanese Australian woman, about 35 years old, who grew up in Bankstown. She has a quintessentially Lebanese-Australian accent (called 'Leb-speak' colloquially by Lebanese-Australians). It is 'Arabic-accented English' with different vowel and stop-rhyme patterns than Anglo-Celtic English (Port and Mitleb 1983). The trainee guide, about 28, is a migrant who came from mainland China in her teens. The guides stand in pedestrian space with a plain black uniform, plus microphone and headset. As the tourists arrive they smile broadly, welcome each new arrival and organise take-away coffees. When all 15 are assembled, the head-guide asks us: while we are all still standing, to introduce ourselves, by talking about our ethnic heritage, our favourite food and why we have come on the tour. Both guides listen to each of us in turn intently, and from time to time make self-deprecating jokes as tourists explain how they have multiple ethnic heritages (Scottish and Irish, Filipino and American, Greek and English) and what foods they like. The guides nod, look interested, lean forward, smile, and make listening noises for each and everyone's talk of 'chillis', 'baklava', 'all foods', 'new foods' 'rice' ... . They explain the purpose of the tour, the nature of the tours as a social enterprise and provide demographics on the suburb. The group visibly relaxes as people change their body language and start to smile.

An Australian-Greek woman guide explains that this is the work of 'ice-breaking' – encouraging tourists to share stories, and welcoming them to southwestern Sydney. In essence, the guides have to produce themselves as a 'welcoming body' (Wise 2005: 175) so that the group feels cared for emotionally, socially and physically. This entails voice, race and body skills and in particular smiling and joking (Veijola and Jokinen 2008). The guides have to produce this 'welcoming body' whilst inhabiting racialized bodies, even in some cases to-be-feared bodies at a time of intense Islamophobia and xenophobia in Australia (Ahmed 2012). Moreover, the pedestrian space outside the railway station in which the guides welcome us, is represented in the media as dangerous and feared as being a hotspot for violence, especially at night.

But racialized bodies are not necessarily seen as 'welcoming' and so performing friendliness when you are from backgrounds that are not seen to be very welcoming, or indeed welcome in Australia, requires particular kinds of emotional techniques. Amanda Wise discusses how elderly, white long-term residents talked about how they perceived the bodies of Chinese shopkeepers as unwelcoming because they did not greet them in the same way that white Anglo-Celtic shopkeepers would do: 'In this case, a welcoming body is expected to display emotions such as pleasure and interest; to signal a 'pleased to see you' (2010: 925). Being seen as friendly is unevenly distributed by race (Ahmed 2013; Tolia-Kelly 2006). Racialized bodies such as those belonging to Muslims are marked as sources of fear or hate (Tolia-Kelly 2006).

The guides are aware that part of their caring work is enabling white tourists to overcome their fears. An Australian-Greek woman guide explains that the tourists need 'someone to ease you into the area. And that way it might enable them to come back. They'll take a different perspective on it. And they'll be quite happy to come back and shop again'. Indeed a repeated theme from the guides was how fearful the tourists can feel because of the racist stereotypes reproduced by the media, histories of racial encounters, and racialized bodies that remind them of tensions, intensities of feeling, even perhaps the 'tempestuous forces' of interracial encounters (Tolia-Kelly and Crang 2010: 2309. See also Ahmed 2012). In particular, guides told us that tourists are scared of the imagined crime and violence in the region. Some tourists confirmed this in conversations with us. As a result, an important part of the guides' work is to emphasize how safe the region is, how friendly and generous the shopkeepers and local residents are. On one occasion we heard a guide using humour to alleviate such fear, joking with the tourists they can see that they do not need to wear bullet-proof vests in Bankstown as it is safe and friendly.

A repeated motif in our interviews was that tourists were afraid to leave their cars in the suburbs in which the tours take place. A few tourists we spoke to admitted they worried about their cars being stolen. An Australian-Greek woman guide explained: 'A lot of people that come on these tours probably don't come across a lot of people with different nationalities. People come to Lakemba completely scared and worried. Like, this lady came and she told me: is it all right to leave my car here?' Part of the guides' caring work then is assuaging the fear of the tourists. We observed they do this in a number of ways, including using humour to relax the group, referring to shopkeepers by their names and in some cases calling them Uncles and encouraging us to enjoy the food and the streets. Whilst some guides might gently tease the tourists about their views on safety, none of them directly challenged them on their racist or sensationalist views about the region in which the guides live and work. This suggests an extra dimension to the emotional labour of the guides in line with the 'extraordinary emotional restraint' that racialized workers have to produce in the face of racism (Wilkins 2012: 34. See also Froyum 2013; Mirchandani 2003). This theme of emotional restraint in the face of racism is exemplified in the following quote from an Australian-Egyptian woman guide who is also Muslim and wears a hijab or headscarf that covers her hair and neck.

> I'm telling them information about Islam and Muslims, and behaviour in Ramadan. But I'm giving it in a way that is fun and acceptable to them. They've probably never had the opportunity to gain this knowledge ... firsthand ... I remember the first time I went on a tour ... This lady ... she said: "how many kids do you have?" I said: "I have three daughters and one boy". She said: "Are you going to force your kids to wear the scarf?" I said: "I have no idea what kind of books you have been reading about Muslims; but believe me, I never force my kids to do anything.

The guide makes it clear that information-giving about Islam is not straightforward. Even though the tourists have chosen to do a tour on Middle-Eastern food, she still has to censor what and how she talks. She also has to contend with a tourist's racist question posed in a direct and personal way. Research on racist abuse in service-work stresses how emotionally draining hearing and having to respond to racial abuse is, leaving service-workers feeling anxious, humiliated and angry. They are required to hostess whilst at the same time contain the affective pressures and intense bodily impressions which Lobo (2014) argues can destabilize racially minoritized women and men.

During our observations we heard other racist comments and questions by tourists and saw tourists grimacing when guides explained what foods we would be tasting, or when they tried particular foods. The guides treated these with patience and good-will, helping the tourists to find ways to change their bodily habits, sense of smell and taste, idea of good manners. In so doing, they laboured to enable tourists to extend their multicultural senses and bodies.

Responding to racism is emotionally intense and not seen as part of good customer service. As Veijola and Valtonen (2007) note, the presence of customer feedback sheets structures how guides act. This is exemplified by this next excerpt taken from our fieldnotes on a 'feasting after fasting' food tour in the Muslim month of Ramadan. This tour was designed to 'bring people together over the dinner table and enable a greater understanding of different cultures and religions'; according to the Taste Tours manager (Jones 2012: np). The manager of the tour explained in a local paper that 'Ramadan is the perfect opportunity to demystify Islam a little bit for the people of Sydney by giving them a change to experience the food and traditions accompanied by a local guide' (ibid.).

The tour started with a meal in a Pakistani-Indian restaurant with two Muslim women guides – one from Pakistan and the other from Egypt – explaining certain food and religious customs; the tour continued with visits to shops and finally coffee in a Middle-Eastern café with a large tent in the back yard. The tour started with a breaking of the fast, followed by the meal with typical dishes from the Indian sub-continent and the Middle East made for Ramadan. This excerpt illustrates the intricate and extensive caring work of the guides:

> At the end of the shopping after dinner, the guides marshalled the group of twelve tourists – mainly white, two Lebanese, one Black American – through a small, crowded Middle-Eastern coffee shop to a marquee tent in the backyard. They had worked hard in the restaurant in front of bemused local residents to relax us all and to explain the meanings of the breaking of the fast, describe the foods we were eating, outline patiently how Ramadan rituals varied between them, visit us round the large table and show us how to eat the different courses. It was the first time such a tour had been run and the Tours manager was present. In the tent, it was warm, hectic, with about 25 Middle-Eastern men in small groups drinking Arabic coffee, sitting round small tables, talking Arabic and laughing and smoking hubbly-bubbly (water-pipe). We seated ourselves higgly-piggly around different tables, a little hesitantly as we weren't sure what was going to happen next. Eventually tea and coffees came and Middle-Eastern sweets on large trays. The two women guides were visibly tired but smiled at us, worked hard to find us seats in the tent. It was late. And they were still checking that we had got our drinks, liaising with the waiter to order special requests and encouraging us to eat. After all this, they then asked us to complete the lengthy feedback forms, providing biros and explaining how helpful it was to them. People had not stopped drinking and eating but tried to balance the forms on the small round coffee tables crowded with cups and sweets. It was dark and noisy, so difficult to write. We didn't complete ours as we were researching but one of the guides was insistent that it was useful information and she would really like us to do it. Finally, she took the completed forms to the Taste Tours manager and they had a quick scan. She looked slightly nervous. But it seemed like the evaluations were positive by some gentle nodding and low-key smiles.

We were surprised the Ramadan dinner finished with the completion of the forms. We and other tourists were less than keen to complete the forms. It felt like an intrusion on what had been a sociable, convivial if a little strained evening. The evaluation form was extensive and detailed with 24 questions with 5-likert-point scale with a third of the questions focused on marketing, a third on demographic information about the tourists and a third on feedback on the guides and the tours. The names of the guides and the tour were at the top of the first page. Whilst Taste Tours is badged as social enterprise designed to do cultural-bridging work, it is the tourists who are asked to judge the success of the tours. As a result, guides spend energy, time and skill on anticipating customers' needs, a central part of hostessing work.

The Benevolent Society values the tours in relation to their reception on tourists –and them feeling satisfied and 'well-treated'. Hostessing academics argue that this takes away the autonomy of service workers in determining the quality of their work. Hage (1997) notes white middle-class, cosmo-multiculturalists see themselves as the ones with the sensitivity, knowledge and care to adjudicate what constitutes authentic ethnic food. On Taste Tours, they are being asked too to evaluate the racialized caring femininity of the guides. This can be seen as a way in which 'colonial judgements' as opposed to local community judgements are being prioritised (Heldke 2003: 15).

This next quotation underlines the pressure this adjudication creates; an Australian-Maltese woman guide explains:

> I'm extremely emotionally attached to this. I can't help it really because when you're a creative person and you put so much of yourself into something you're putting it out there for random strangers. People who are actually into food. You're putting it out there for them to judge. Not only that; you're putting the future of Taste Tours on the line as well. So there's a huge amount of responsibility that I feel.

The guide 'others' the tourists when she refers to them as strangers. She describes how the emotional warmth on tours is a form of labour, not the result of friendship. She also emphasizes how her caring work extends to include the reputation of the social enterprise. As discussed in the service-work literature, customers are positioned as judge and jury, reproducing asymmetrical power relations in which the guides are not seen as foodie experts but as servers and 'locals'. On Taste Tours, this sense of deference and subservience is amplified through the social enterprise aims and connotations of benevolence. This comes through strongly in the next quote from the Australian-Maltese guide:

> They expect when you're handing things out, the napkin should be there, the hand sanitizer should be there, everything should be paid for. They have an expectation – you can tell that they have an expectation after having done tours that expectation is there. So you're almost like a server to them. You're almost like a waiter or a waitress to them: who is there to provide this experience for them. Sort of like an airline hostess.

Explicitly echoing the term hostessing here, the guide understands the hierarchy of guiding work. Like many service workers, she knows that caring service-work is complex but devalued.

Conclusion

In this chapter we have examined the caring work undertaken by migrant Australian women tour guides on Taste Tours, an ethnic neighbourhood food-tourism social enterprise, run by The Benevolent Society. We explore their caring work through the analytic categories of emotional labour and hostessing because the literature on emotional labour values the complex skills of caring work and places their performance within a larger context of the service economy, epitomised by tourism. Moreover, the analytical categories foreground gender, the blurring of the domestic and work, and ongoing inequalities in relation to caring and skill in tourism. They help us highlight one of the forms of care on Taste Tours. This literature, however, has under-researched the racialization of emotional labour and hostessing, which has to be explored in the context of The Benevolent Society, southwestern Sydney and the work of the tour guides. In particular, we argue that this racialized context creates particular 'audience-effects' (Adkins 2005; Jokinen and Veijola 2012; Veijola 2009) and 'emotional impressions' (Ahmed 2012; Lobo 2014) with, and against which, the guides have to work.

In their introduction to this book, Lavis, Abbots and Attala ask what relationships are produced through care and eating, and how these intervene in individual bodies and shape particular forms of eating. In analysing the racialized emotional labour of tour guides, we show how hostess-tourist relations in this context, shape the bodies of the workers as they try to please, welcome and relax the tourists, and manage racialized intensities and impressions. At the same time, these relationships intervene in the bodies of the tourists as they learn to taste, smell and eat different foods and walk through racialized spaces. We discuss how the guides through their 'hostessing' enable the tourists to experience warm relations with them and the local residents and to feel safe when they may have racist assumptions or feelings about the guides and the region. Furthermore, tourists may be curious about eating different foods and being in the midst of racialized spaces but their bodies may betray them in feeling disgust, stopping them from eating the Other with the vigour they wished (Longhurst, Ho and Johnston 2008). Or they may want to eat particular 'ethnic' foods but not have the know-how. The guides respond to these situations, caring for them by sharing stories, through ethnic feeding work and eating techniques, being patient and attentive, undertaking fear-assuaging work and enabling tourists to develop 'multicultural senses, relations and bodies'.

In addition to caring for the tourists, the guides work hard to care for the work of The Benevolent Society and the representation of southwestern Sydney and its residents. To produce the 'cared for' tourist, the guides have to suppress any anger and frustration about racism. Whilst in asymmetrical power, bodily and emotional relations of the service encounter, the guides use their agency to offer alternative views of the region, their expertise and the lives of the locals to counter racist and racialized assumptions the tourists may hold (Bunten 2011, 2013).

Furthermore, the tours are not straightforwardly commercial tourism but run as a social enterprise by a large charity with Christian roots. The tourists are positioned as benefactors with local residents and guides seen as grateful recipients in need of their help through the framing of the tours as 'eating for a good cause'. Indeed, the guides commence the tours begin by reminding everyone that they are on a social enterprise. As part of this, the guides were 'othered' on the webpage, at the time of our research, as housewives and mothers who cook for love, rather than as professionals with postgraduate qualifications. Hence, on Taste Tours, eating the Other is constructed as caring for the Other.

The caring agenda (Lavis et al., this volume) of The Benevolent Society is to use the guides' work as part of their community-building initiatives in the region, which includes repairing 'cultural and intergenerational divides'. The Benevolent Society benefits from the expertise of the guides, including their femininity and ethnicity as workplace 'assets' and their caring practices, service-producing bodies and ethnic feeding work as resources. At the same time, it does not provide the material, cultural or social resources with which the tours can acknowledge the wider context of colonial racialized relations, inequalities and racism. This is possible, as Emily Drew's (2011) work on anti-racist tourism shows. As Ahmed puts it: 'the desire to feel good or better can involve the erasure of relations of violence covering them over so can there can be a return to national pride' (2012: 197). Indeed, we can say that the sophisticated caring work of the Other produces white benevolence.

In sum, Taste Tours can be understood as a form of economic, cultural and social production. Capitalism has always exploited women's emotional labour and caring work in producing life but scholars suggest there is 'unprecedented intensification of appropriating women, femininity and women's work in the global labour market' (Veijola and Jokinen 2008: 121). The work of the guides helps sustain the life of multiculturalism in the face of racism, xenophobia and Islamophobia. It is what we call 'multiculturalism-as-work': producing relations, bodies and emotions which enable people to live together among difference, and often performed by migrant women in unpaid labour or undervalued paid labour. More concisely, the tourists learn to care for the Other through the Other caring for them.

Acknowledgements

We would like to thank everyone at Taste Tours and the Benevolent Society for giving us their time and access to the project.

References

Adkins, L. 2005. The new economy, property and personhood. *Theory, Culture & Society*, 22(1), 111-30.

Ahmed, S. 2002. *Strange Encounters: Embodied Others in Post-Coloniality.* London: Routledge.

Ahmed, S. 2004a. Affective economies. *Social Text*, 22(2), 117-39.

Ahmed, S. 2004b. Collective feelings or, the impressions left by others. *Theory, Culture & Society*, 21(2), 25-42.

Ahmed, S. 2012. *The Cultural Politics of Emotion.* London: Routledge.

Bolton, S.C. 2009. Getting to the heart of the emotional labour process: A reply to Brook. *Work, Employment & Society*, 23(3), 549-60.

Bolton, S.C. and Houlihan, M. 2005. The (mis) representation of customer service. *Work, Employment & Society*, 19(4), 685-703.

Bunten, A. 2008. Sharing culture or selling out? *American Ethnologist*, 35(3), 380-95.

Charmaz, K. 2014. *Constructing Grounded Theory.* London: Sage.

Clarke, G. 2013. *The Roots of Benevolence: Christian Ideals and Social Benefit.* http://www.abc.net.au/religion/articles/2013/05/08/3754498.htm [accessed: 1 March 2013].

Cohen, E. 1985. The Tourist Guide: The origins, structure and dynamics of a role. *Annals of Tourism Research*, 12(1), 5-29.

Collins, J. 2009. Sydney's Cronulla riots: The context and implications, in *Lines in the Sand*, edited by G. Noble. Sydney: Institute of Criminology Press, 27-43.

Conforti, J. 1996. Ghettos as tourism attractions. *Annals of Tourism Research*, 23(4), 830-42.

Crang, P. 1997. Performing the tourist product, in *Touring Cultures: Transformations of Travel and Theory*, edited by C. Rojek and J. Urry. London: Routledge, 137-54.

Duffy, M. 2007. Doing the dirty work: Gender, race, and reproductive labor in Historical Perspective. *Gender & Society*, 21(3), 313-36.

Duruz, J. 2010. Floating food: Eating 'Asia' in kitchens of the diaspora. *Emotion, Space and Society*, 3(1), 45-49.

Dreher, T. 2006. From cobra grubs to dragons: Negotiating the politics of representation in cultural research. *Cultural Studies Review*, 12(2), 90-106.

Emerson, R.M. 2001. *Contemporary Field Research: Perspectives and Formulations.* Prospect Heights, IL: Waveland Press.

Flowers, R. and Swan, E. 2012. Eating the Asian Other? Pedagogies of food multiculturalism in Australia. *PORTAL Journal of Multidisciplinary International Studies*, 9(2), 1-30.

Flowers, R. and Swan, E. In press 2015. Potatoes in the rice cooker: Family food pedagogies, bodily memories, meal-time senses and racial practices, in *Food Pedagogies*, edited by R. Flowers and E. Swan. Farnham: Ashgate.

Froyum, C. 2013. 'For the betterment of kids who look like me': Professional emotional labour as a racial project. *Ethnic and Racial Studies*, 36(6), 1070-89.

Glaser, J. 1994. Conflicting loyalties: Beneficence – love within limits, in *Theological Analyses of the Clinical Encounter*, edited by G. McKenny and J. Sande. Dordrecht: Kluwer, 109-32.

Gray, A. 2003. Enterprising femininity: New modes of work and subjectivity. *European Journal of Cultural Studies*, 6(4), 489-506.

Gunew, S. 1993. *Against multiculturalism*: Rhetorical images in Multiculturalism, Difference and Postmodernism, in *Multiculturalism, Difference and Postmodernism*, edited by G.L. Clark, D. Forbes and R. Francis. Melbourne: Longman Cheshire, 38-53.

Gunaratnam, Y. and Lewis, G. 2001. Racialising emotional labour and emotionalising racialised labour: Anger, fear and shame in social welfare. *Journal of Social Work Practice*, 15(2), 131-48.

Hage, G. 1997. At home in the entrails of the West: Multiculturalism, ethnic food and migrant home-building, in *Home/world: Space, Community and Marginality in Sydney's West*, edited by H. Grace, G. Hage, L. Johnson, J. Langsworth and M. Symonds, Pluto, Annandale, 99-153.

Hage, Ghassan, April 23, 2008. Roots will be with you always. *The Australian Newspaper* [online]. Available at: http://www.theaustralian.com.au/ higher-education/appointments/rootswill-be-with-you-always/story-e6frgckf-1111116133196 [accessed: 17 March 2013].

Haugh, H. 2005. A research agenda for social entrepreneurship. *Social Enterprise Journal*, 1(1), 1-12.

Heldke, L. 2003. *Exotic Appetites: Ruminations of a Food Adventurer*. London: Routledge.

Highmore, B. 2008. Alimentary agents: Food, cultural theory and multiculturalism. *Journal of Intercultural Studies*, 29(4), 381-98.

hooks, b. 1992. Eating the Other, in *Black Looks: Race and Representation*. Boston, MA: South End Press, 21-39.

Jack, G. and Phipps, A.M. 2005. *Tourism and Intercultural Exchange: Why Tourism Matters* (No. 4). Bristol: Channel View Publications.

Jackson, P. 1999. Consumption and identity: The cultural politics of shopping. *European Planning Studies*, 7(1), 25-39.

Jakubowicz, A. and Ho, C. (eds). 2014. *'For Those Who've Come Across the Seas ... ': Australian Multicultural Theory, Policy and Practice*. Sydney: Anthem Press.

Johnston, L. and Longhurst, R. 2012. Embodied geographies of food, belonging and hope in multicultural Hamilton, Aotearoa New Zealand. *Geoforum*, 43(2), 325-31.

Jokinen, E. and Veijola, S. 2012. Time to hostess. *Real Tourism: Practice, Care, and Politics in Contemporary Travel Culture*, 26, 38-70.

Jones, G. 2012. Ramadan food tours shed light on Islam, *Daily Telegraph*, August 15, [online]. Available at: http://www.dailytelegraph.com.au/ramadan-food-tours-shed-light-on-islam/story-e6freuy9-226450367270?nk=38e2fe5fb87cf0 430b9a1fb790aa3a28 [accessed: 15 March 2013].

Lobo, M. 2014. Affective energies: Sensory bodies on the beach in Darwin, Australia. *Emotion, Space and Society*, 12, 101-9.

Longhurst, R., Ho, E. and Johnston, L. 2008. Using 'the body' as an 'instrument of research': Kimch'i and pavlova. *Area*, 40(2), 208-17.

Lovell, T. 2000. Thinking feminism with and against Bourdieu. *Feminist theory*, 1(1), 11-32.

Macdonald, C.L. and Sirianni, C. (eds). 1996. *Working in the Service Society*. Philadelphia, PA: Temple University Press.

Michaux, A. 2010. Integrating knowledge in service delivery-land: A view from The Benevolent Society, in *Bridging the 'Know-Do' Gap: Knowledge Brokering to Improve Child Wellbeing*, edited by G. Bammer, A. Michaux, and A. Sanson. Canberra: ANUE Press, 12-36.

Mirchandani, K. 2003. Challenging racial silences in studies of emotion work: Contributions from anti-racist feminist theory. *Organization Studies*, 24(5), 721-42.

Mirchandani, K. 2012. *Phone Clones: Authenticity Work in the Transnational Service Economy*. New York: Cornell University Press.

Molz, J.G. 2007. Eating difference: The cosmopolitan mobilities of culinary tourism. *Space and Culture*, 10(1), 77-93.

Narayan, U. 1997. *Dislocating Cultures: Identities, Traditions, and Third World Feminism*. London: Routledge.

Noble, G. 2009. Where the bloody hell are we?, in *Lines in the Sand*, edited by G. Noble. Sydney: Institute of Criminology Press, 1-22.

Poynting, S., Noble, G., Tabar, G. and Collins, J. 2004. *Bin Laden in the Suburbs: Criminalising the Arab Other*. Sydney: Sydney Institute of Criminology.

Probyn, E. 2000. *Carnal Appetites: Foodsexidentities*. Sydney: Psychology Press.

Ramos-Zayas, A.Y. 2012. *Street Therapists: Race, Affect, and Neoliberal Personhood in Latino Newark*. Chicago, IL: University of Chicago Press.

Riggs, D. 2004. *Constructing the National Good: Howard and the Rhetoric of Benevolence*. Paper at Australasian Political Studies Association Conference, University of Adelaide.

Salazar, N.B. 2008. 'Enough stories!' Asian tourism redefining the roles of Asian tour guides. *Civilisations*, 57(1/2), 207-22.

Santos, C., Belhassen, Y. and Caton, K. 2008. Re-imagining Chinatown: An analysis of tourism discourse. *Tourism Management*, 29(5), 1002-12.

Shan, H. 2012. Learning to 'fit in': The emotional work of Chinese immigrants in Canadian engineering workplaces. *Journal of Workplace Learning*, 24(5), 351-64.

Sheller, M. 2003. *Consuming the Caribbean: From Arawaks to Zombies*. London: Routledge.

Sheridan, S. 2000. Eating the Other: Food and cultural difference in the Australian Women's Weekly in the 1960s. *Journal of Intercultural Studies*, 21(3), 319-29.

Skeggs, B. 2004. Context and background: Pierre Bourdieu's analysis of class, gender and sexuality. *The Sociological Review*, 52(2), 19-33.

Skinner, J. and Theodossopoulos, D. (eds). 2011. *Great Expectations: Imagination and Anticipation in Tourism* (Vol. 34). Cambridge: Berghahn Books.

Swan, E. 2008. 'You make me feel like a woman': Therapeutic cultures and the contagion of femininity. *Gender, Work & Organization*, 15(1), 88-107.

The Benevolent Society 2011 [online]. Available at: http://www.benevolent.org.au/think/doing--things--differently/taste--food--tours [accessed: 14 April 2013].

The Benevolent Society 2014. *Our Story* [online]. Available at: http://www.benevolent.org.au/about/celebrating--200--years [accessed: 5 August 2013].

Tolia-Kelly, D.P. 2006. Affect – an ethnocentric encounter? Exploring the 'universalist'imperative of emotional/affectual geographies. *Area*, 38(2), 213-17.

Tolia-Kelly, D.P. and Crang, M. 2010. Affect, race, and identities. *Environment and Planning A*, 42(10), 2309-14.

Valkonen, J. 2009. Acting in nature: Service events and agency in wilderness guiding. *Tourist Studies*, 9(2), 164-80.

Valtonen, A. 2009. Small tourism firms as agents of critical knowledge. *Tourist Studies*, 9(2), 127-43.

Veijola, S. and Valtonen, A. 2007. The body in tourism industry. *Tourism and Gender: Embodiment, Sensuality and Experience*. Oxford: CABI, 13-31.

Veijola, S. and Jokinen, E. 2005. Hostessing, gender and work, paper presented at the special session: *Hostesses of the World: Sexuality, Power and Gender*, 37th International Conference of the IIS, Stockholm, 5-9 July.

Veijola, S. and Jokinen, E. 2008. Towards a hostessing society? Mobile arrangements of gender and labour. *NORA—Nordic Journal of Feminist and Gender Research*, 16(3), 166-81.

Veijola, S. 2009a. Introduction: Tourism as work. *Tourist Studies*, 9(2), 83-7.

Veijola, S. 2009b. Gender as work in the tourism industry. *Tourist studies*, 9(2), 109-26.

White, P. 2004. *Media Savages Lebanese-Australian Youth* [online]. Available at: http://www.onlineopinion.com.au [accessed: 10 February 2014].

Wilkins, A. 2012. 'Not out to start a revolution': Race, gender, and emotional restraint among black university men. *Journal of Contemporary Ethnography*, 41(1), 34-65.

Wingfield, A.H. 2010. Are some emotions marked 'whites only'? Racialised feeling rules in professional workplaces. *Social Problems*, 57(2), 251-68.

Wong, J.Y. and Wang, C.H. 2009. Emotional labor of the tour leaders: An exploratory study. *Tourism Management*, 30(2), 249-59.

Wise, A. 2005. Hope and belonging in a multicultural suburb. *Journal of Intercultural Studies*, 26(1-2), 171-86.

Wise, A. 2010. Sensuous multiculturalism: Emotional landscapes of inter-ethnic living in Australian suburbia. *Journal of Ethnic and Migration Studies*, 36(6), 917-37.

Wise, A. and Velayutham, A. (eds) 2009. *Everyday Multiculturalism*. Basingstoke: Palgrave Macmillan.

Chapter 2

Is Sharing Caring? Social Media and Discourses of Healthful Eating

Signe Rousseau

Dear journalist. Please spare me ur simplistic soundbite nutrition msgs. Nutrition & food are not black & white issues.[1]

Social media allow and encourage everyone with access to the Internet to have a voice. These networking platforms are therefore the sites in which some of the most dynamic conversations take place and strongest communities are forged in our present 'digital age'. Given our appetite for thinking about eating, moreover, it is perhaps inevitable that food has been one of the fastest growing topics on platforms like Twitter and Pinterest, where sharing, I argue, has become a shorthand for caring about what you eat. But social media also provide spaces which are fruitful for setting up false dichotomies between 'good', 'nurturing' and 'safe' foods and those that are products of scientific interventions (for example GMOs and the recent world-first 'test tube' burger), thought to be harmful to the environment and to healthy bodies. Inasmuch as they bring people together, then, social media can equally contribute to producing fractious and fractured communities that ultimately obstruct productive conversations about how best to care for ourselves, for our families, and for the planet.

This chapter focuses chiefly on Twitter as a space for debating topical issues related to health and eating. Following a brief overview of some of the existing research on social media, it considers three key subject areas which are particularly relevant to a paradigm of care and, more specifically, to the social dynamics embedded in the question of why (some) people care about what others eat. The first of these is scientifically engineered food, where caring most obviously manifests as *scaring*, typically by appeal to the naturalistic fallacy. Second are the discourses around obesity and other 'lifestyle diseases', where personal choices are most keenly scrutinized, critiqued, and in some cases leveraged as active resistance against a widespread moralizing trend, as in the case of the #notyourgoodfatty hashtag. The final – and arguably key – issue is that of authority, or of who has the (ostensible) right to make pronouncements and prescriptions about how others (ought to) eat. The question of authority is of course closely related to the examples of both scientifically-modified foods and obesity, but all three combine

---

1   Tweeted by @Inglesdietitian on 17 April 2014, https://twitter.com/InglesDietitian/status/456585781130174464.

to demonstrate how the traditional hierarchies of food brokers (those informing and governing others' food choices) and eaters (those making food choices) are not necessarily disturbed *by* social media, but disturbances to which are made all the more visible *through* social media.[2] In short, these relatively new technological tools are useful for exposing existing hierarchies of careful eating, particularly as those structures are challenged by new and emerging sites of authority.

It should be emphasized from the outset that it is not my contention that social media platforms are exclusive agents in disrupting conventional notions of care and expertise. It is, rather, to suggest that the technology behind social media can contribute a precipitating agency to the already-fraught arena of discourses around what is 'good' and 'proper' when it comes to how and what to eat. Not only would the former grant too much agency to a tool designed and operated by people, but it would also ignore the extent to which social media are not extrinsic to everyday life. Quite the opposite; even if at times put in service of explicitly *anti*-social behaviours, social media have quickly become intrinsic to the basic (but by no means easy) business of managing our own – and others' – lives.

Prosumption, Produsage, and Mediated Mobilism

Often touted as a key characteristic of social media is the idea of 'prosumption', or the conflation of production and consumption (Rousseau 2012b). Prosumption describes the fact that we no longer merely consume, but also produce information every time we partake in social media activity, for example by tweeting, updating a Facebook status, penning or commenting on a blog post, to name just a few of the now myriad ways that we get involved. Some, like sociologists George Ritzer[3] and Nathan Jurgenson, argue that capitalist economies have always been informed by the twin priorities of production and consumption (for example in fast food restaurants where patrons have to clean up after themselves by throwing away containers and any uneaten food, thereby becoming part of the production chain), but that technologies such as social networking sites simply foreground and enhance the 'means of prosumption' in a way that is less exploitative and ultimately more enjoyable (Ritzer and Jurgenson 2010: 19). Given that prosumption is therefore more 'evolutionary' than 'revolutionary' (where a site like Amazon is, for instance, just a 'logical extension' of physical shopping malls), Ritzer cautions against 'operating with a dualistic sense of the material and digital worlds' as the two are now largely indistinguishable, and the distinctions increasingly meaningless (Ritzer 2014: 10. See also Ritzer et al. 2012). Media scholar Axel Bruns adds a further dimension of appropriation with his model of 'produser',

---

2   My thanks to my husband Jacques Rousseau for helping to articulate this point.

3   Ritzer is perhaps best known for the theory of McDonalidzation – characterized by the four priorities of efficiency, calculability, predictability, and control – as a feature of modern globalization.

which prioritizes our roles as users rather than consumers of information (Bruns 2008). This is in keeping with active audience theorists such as Michel de Certeau and John Fiske who in the 1980s contributed to destabilizing the model of 'the' homogeneous media pitted against a similarly homogeneous mass of passive consumers (Rousseau 2012a: 59).

Focused more on the intersection between use(r)s and the technology itself is work that examines the appropriation process, or how new technologies are 'domesticated', Maren Hartmann suggests the notion of 'mediated mobilism' to describe the convergence of mobile media with the 'consequences of increased fluctuation, mobilization, and mobility' among users (Hartmann 2013: 46). This 'double articulation' of technology and content is similarly explored by Stine Lomborg, who proposes that social media could more usefully be considered as 'communicative genres', the difference being that a medium exhibits 'technical-material features' whereas genres are more about 'communicative conventions and expectations' (Lomborg 2011: 58). She does, however, point out that some media features are also 'socially negotiated', so the distinction is by no means failsafe, with Twitter as a case in point: 'The microblog is an example of a communicative genre at work across various media platforms, framed in the interplay between the Internet and the mobile phone as communication media' (ibid.: 60).

The evolution – and to some extent, therefore, instability – of theories about social media are perhaps appropriate to the fluctuations of the media (or genres, per Lomborg) themselves, understood both in terms of their technical possibilities and how – and for what purposes – they are used. As Lomborg also points out, while Twitter was not originally designed for conversation,

> users themselves started having conversations and to spread each other's tweets, resulting in, for instance, the addressivity function of the @ sign and the RT (retweet) function being embedded over time (...). By making changes at the software level, Twitter has sought to adjust the service to users' needs and practices. (ibid.: 67)

It is no doubt the case that most social networking sites would justify their continuous re-designs and updates as being in the interests of users' needs and practices. Yet the fact that neither the technology nor its purpose is static or singular should also serve as a caution about the limitations of theory. Whether we call ourselves (and others) prosumers, produsers, or agents – possibly even victims – of 'mediated mobilism', conversations (and disagreements) on social media platforms demonstrate that inasmuch as food and eating can, as the editors explain in their introduction to this volume, produce otherness and create social distance just as much as it can integrate and dissolve social boundaries, so can just *talking* about food and eating.

Cultured Beef

On August 15, 2013, the world's first 'test tube' burger was cooked and tasted in a live broadcast, with #culturedbeef trending on Twitter for the hour or so of the proceedings. Made possible by funding (to the tune of $325,000) by Sergey Brin, co-founder of Google, the event provided an excellent sketch of the intersections between food, science, popular culture and the twin poles of care and disgust. It featured a (typically affordable) iconic, familiar, form of comfort food, but in an (expensive) unfamiliar, futuristic guise. It was simultaneously an imaginary 'Frankenfood' and reportedly mundane in its blandness (Brewster 2013). Staged for the camera, it was at once a public performance, and also a virtual peek into the world of laboratory scientists, where most of us never venture. With a live audience of journalists, and a virtual audience of anyone with an Internet connection, its format straddled the tropes of entertainment, education and news. It was an exclusive event with a massive guest list. The spectacle enacted the crossover between the proverbial high and low brow cultures of food, and instantly became part of a dynamic global conversation.

This conversation is by no means new, having been sustained in various guises over several decades at least since the inauguration of the Green Revolution pioneered by Nobel Laureate Norman Borlaug.[4] It is a conversation regularly punctuated by high profile institutional involvements and pronouncements and, above all, shaped by controversy, for example Greenpeace's ongoing campaign against the genetically modified 'golden rice'[5] in a move that has been condemned as a 'crime against humanity' (Connor 2014: np).[6] Unhindered by a limit of 140 characters, these polarized positions migrate with remarkable ease to a platform like Twitter:

> @sexyfoodtherapy This is how I feel about #GMOs. #frankenfood #junkfood #jerf #audreyhepburn #middlefinger #fckyou … [accompanied by an Instagrammed photograph of Audrey Hepburn with her middle finger raised][7]

---

4   Borlaug is also known as the 'man who saved a billion lives' after developing and introducing high-yielding and disease-resistant crop varieties to famine-vulnerable areas like Asia, Africa and South America (AP 2009).

5   'Golden rice' was developed to address Vitamin A deficiencies, estimated to contribute to childhood blindness and to the deaths of millions of children annually (Harmon 2013).

6   Other recent controversies include the 'Prop 37' and 'I-522' campaigns for labelling of genetically modified (GM) foods in the states of California and Washington, respectively. During these campaigns, environmental activist Mark Lynas, famously an early opponent of GMOs, publicly pronounced that he had changed his mind, and is now a firm supporter of genetic modification.

7   11 April 2014, https://twitter.com/sexyfoodtherapy/status/454475658702635009.

@Jennifur_Rainey: Disgusting, Creepy & Gross! #InvitroMeat now they are growing meat in labs http://en.wikipedia.org/wiki/In_vitro_meat … In-Vitro meats http://www.futurefood.org/in-vitro-meat/index_en.php …[8]

The Twitter account @invitromeat, meanwhile, was founded by '[T]wo students from Beckmans College of Design, searching for a GOOD argument against In Vitro Meat', as their Twitter profile puts it. The fact that their last (re)tweet was in October 2011[9] suggests that their endeavour was unsuccessful.

The key difference between the longer ongoing conversations about the intersections between science and food, like those related to genetic modification, and the more recent one about cultured beef and the 'lab-grown' burger is, as one group of writers summarizes it, that 'the cells [in cultured meat] are generated through a tissue culture and cloning process that creates entirely new meat cells, rather than modifying existing cells' (Humes, Runquist and Weldon 2014). This distinction, which would allow (at least theoretically, considering the at-present prohibitive cost factor) for meat to be produced without harming animals or the environment, could be marshalled to generate a new set of ethical food parameters, argues the philosopher Julian Baggini (2013). But there is stronger evidence for a continued appeal to the naturalistic fallacy (in which anything from nature is considered 'good', and anything not is therefore 'bad' and probably unsafe), and to extremism over nuance:

> The belief that we have to choose between a food system that is over-dependent on technology and one that is more in harmony with nature rests on the assumption that there is a neat moral and conceptual contrast between 'natural' and 'artificial', and that this lines up neatly with the distinction between 'good' and 'bad'. If IVM [in vitro meat] is the greenest, most animal-friendly meat, yet it is even more artificial than a pitiful, intensively reared broiler chicken, then no one can maintain the fantasy that bucolic nature has a monopoly on good, ethical food … . IVM is just the most recent, vivid example of how our desire for the natural, traditional and aesthetically appealing food can clash with the value we place on animal welfare, environmental sustainability and the humane imperative to feed the whole world well. Almost all the coverage of IVM has glossed over this pluralism, presenting commentators as either for or against, period. (Baggini 2013: np)

Somewhat ironically in an environment characterized by the mobility and fluctuations that generate 'mediated mobilism', this lack of pluralism is arguably part of what could be termed the current 'foodie zeitgeist'. This is the broader climate that both hosts and, to some extent, governs how people think about how and what to eat. It is the sentiment of leading food broker Michael Pollan,

---

8   4 October 2011, https://twitter.com/Jennyfur_Rainey/status/121259154844299266.
9   14 October 2011, https://twitter.com/invitromeat/status/124835784418263041.

whose perceived authority is reflected in one writer's description of him as the 'High priest of American Food' (Kandil 2013), and whose 2013 book *Cooked* is summarized by one reviewer:

> Put simply, "good" transformations of the elemental world are premodern and elemental, while "bad" ones are industrial and high tech … . In the final analysis, the book serves forth a resolutely humanist story of cooking as that which might rescue the author's nation from "abstract" work and engineered food. In response to the felt risks that science and technology pose to the alimentary realm, Pollan works to root his American reader in an *elemental* purpose of cooking: to cultivate human bonds, above all else. (Carruth 2013: np, emphasis in the original)

It is this focus on 'real' food as a fundamentally *humanist* project which frames the issue of industrially engineered food as being much less about scientific literacy and progress than it is about ethics and care – for yourself, for others, and for the planet.

To be sure, as Carolyn Mattick and Brad Allenby put it in their article on 'The Future of Meat' (2014), 'Food is a culturally charged domain, and the technological evolution of meat may well outpace the cultural acceptance of radically new food production technology', adding that focus group studies show that people have a 'negative visceral reaction to the thought of lab-grown meat' (Mattick and Allenby 2014: np). It is, in short, an intuitive rather than evidence-based reaction, and one for which Twitter hashtags like #Frankenfood and #jerf (just eat real food) enact both the 'technical-material features' of the character limitations of microblogging and also the now-solidifying 'communicative conventions and expectations' (Lomborg 2011: 59) of a particular (anti-food-tech) ideological position.[10] By emphasizing a particular use (rather than mere consumption) of information driven by an explicit agenda of instilling fear, this example could also be considered one of the produsage of *scare* in the ostensible service of care. And if there is little evidence of plurality on less space-constrained platforms like blogs and websites, then a social media site like Twitter is even less likely to encourage distinctions from the 'black-and-white, emotionally charged view of agriculture and eating' that one writer (Danovich 2014: np) laments the current 'food movement' as inhabiting: 'Yes, we want more people to get involved in the fight for more transparency, better worker protection, and increased access to good food, but has anyone stopped to wonder what kind of movement we'll have if we only get new members by scaring them into joining?' (ibid.).

One possible answer to that question, and as a concluding consideration for this section, is that it will (and may already) be the kind of movement that is fuelled in

---

10   This is also a good example of what social psychologist Jonathan Haidt has termed the 'emotional dog and its rational tail', by which moral reasoning is 'generated *after* a judgment has been reached' (Haidt 2001: 814, my emphasis).

large part by confirmation bias, or favouring information that supports rather than challenges our existing worldviews. It should be emphasized that the argument here is not that social media *make* us biased, but that filtering mechanisms such as hashtags certainly make it easier to follow and share opinions which may be blinkered or uninformed, and thereby could work to consolidate existing or emergent biases.[11] This scenario is well summarized in a blog post called 'The Terrible Tragedy of the Healthy Eater', which satirizes what happens when you go online to learn how to eat well:

> That really skinny old scientist dude says anything from an animal will give you cancer. But a super-ripped 60 year old with a best-selling diet book says eat more butter with your crispy T-Bone and you'll be just fine as long as you stay away from grains. Great abs beat out the PhD so you end up hanging out on a forum where everyone eats green apples and red meat and talks about how functional and badass parkour is.
>
> You learn that basically, if you ignore civilization and Mark Knopfler music, the last 10,000 years of human development has been one big societal and nutritional cock-up and wheat is entirely to blame. What we all need to do is eat like cave-people. (Strauss 2012: np)

It is to some of those who advocate eating like cave-people, or rather like pre-agricultural hunter-gatherers, that I now turn.

#RealMealRevolution

As scary as they are for some, genetically modified foods represent only a small portion of the industrialized food system that many associate with the arguably scarier phenomenon of a global obesity crisis.[12] The following two sections address some of the ways that public and private health discussions are framed on Twitter, specifically with regard to interventions – including publicly voiced resistance to the perceived need for interventions – as a way to perform care for the self and for others through food choices. Here again we see how traditional hierarchies are made more visible through social media networks, and as they revolve around

---

11   Another way to frame the same mechanism is that social media encourage what Ethan Zuckerman (2008) terms homophily, or 'love of the same', and that many of our activities on the Internet in general take place in what Eli Pariser (2011) calls a 'filter bubble'.

12   It is beyond the scope and purpose of this chapter to rehearse the expansive body of work that deals with obesity as a public health crisis, and whether it merits the moniker of epidemic. See, for example, Gard and Wright (2005), Campos et al. (2006), and LeBesco (2010).

choices that are seemingly private, but with potentially wider public health implications, these discussions around health and weight are particularly fraught with the complexities of authority.

One notable development in the last decade or so is the notion that many of our modern ills – to which obesity and so-called lifestyle ailments like type 2 diabetes and cardiovascular disease belong – are the result of preferring a modern industrial diet (typically high in refined carbohydrates) over eating like our ancestors (the 'cave-people') apparently did (Teicholz 2014).[13] This is the thinking behind diets – or rather new lifestyles as they are often referred to, with the suggestion that this is not a short-term solution focused 'just' on weight loss, but indeed a better way to live a generally healthier life – variously labelled as paleo, low-carb (with echoes of the Atkins diet popular some time ago, and still held up as an important precursor here), or LCHF (low-carbohydrate, high-fat). Some of the most popular US-based authorities are sites like Jimmy Moore's Livin' La Vida Low-Carb (http://livinlavidalowcarb.com/blog/), the Diet Doctor (www. dietdoctor.com, offering "Real Food for Your Health"), and Authority Nutrition, which promises '*the truth* about nutrition' (http://authoritynutrition.com/about/, emphases in the original).

The LCHF movement got a further recent boost when Professor Tim Noakes, the highly rated South African sports scientist who had famously been advocating 'carbo-loading' for marathon runners and other athletes since the publication of his 1985 best-selling *The Lore of Running*, publicly claimed that everything he thought he knew about nutrition had been wrong. He subsequently began to advocate the LCHF diet, particularly for those who are carbohydrate-intolerant and insulin-resistant (both often precursors to and symptoms of type 2 diabetes, which Noakes claims to have developed after a lifetime of eating too many carbohydrates and other 'wrong' foods like those labelled low-fat). In 2013 he co-authored (with two chefs and a nutritionist) a best-selling cookbook called *The Real Meal Revolution*. The LCHF diet is popular enough that it is known locally in South Africa as the Noakes or Banting diet,[14] with restaurants and other eateries offering specialized Noakes or Banting menu options. In April 2014, it was announced (on *Twitter*) that the '1st International Low Carb, High Fat Lifestyle Conference' was scheduled to take place in South Africa, featuring @ProfTimNoakes and @livinlowcarbman (Jimmy Moore).[15]

Common to the narrative and ethos of the Paleo community is the notion not only that we have been eating 'wrongly', but also that we have been duped into doing so by corporate interests that prioritize money and politics over public health

---

13   The question of what our ancestors actually ate, including whether this was 'better' for us, is not without contention either. See, for example, Zuk (2013).

14   William Banting was a British undertaker who was among the first to popularize a low-carbohydrate eating plan through his booklet called *Letter on Corpulence, Addressed to the Public*, published in 1863.

15   27 April 2014, https://twitter.com/HELPdietSA/status/460527433310289920.

(Taubes 2002, 2007). In this scenario, it is the combined efforts of Big Food, Big Ag, and Big Pharma which conspire to make us fat and sick. Part of embracing the lifestyle, therefore, involves nurturing a distrust of what may be termed conventional sites of authority or expertise, like doctors, registered dietitians and government departments tasked with developing nutritional guidelines. A few examples from Noakes's Twitter timeline exemplify the trend:

@ProfTimNoakes: @PastryKeegan The public will decide. In era of social media, public will eventually discover what works for each, independent of "experts"[16]

@ProfTimNoakes: Debate increasingly irrelevant since informed patients now making therapeutic choices for themselves independent of "experts"[17]

@ashman_65: @ProfTimNoakes great response Tim. I have seen many skeptics converted. I no longer trust my doc #lchf[18]

@ProfTimNoakes: Heart Foundations will soon have to answer for contribution to global obesity/diabetes epidemic. http://amzn.to/1gGoVmB [link Nina Teicholz' 2014 book, *The Big Fat Surprise: Why Butter, Meat and Cheese Belong in a Healthy Diet*][19]

@OzParadoxdotcom: Congrats to @garytaubes @ProfTimNoakes @ livinlowcarbman et al. for rebirthing Banting's #LCHF cure, downsizing misery for millions.[20]

These themes are of course not exclusive to Paleo/LCHF/Banting narratives, but belong to a wider trend of responding to various food crises by reinforcing how *little* consumers know, and therefore how little actual control they have over their choices. As Emma-Jayne Abbots and Benjamin Coles put it in the context of 'Horsemeat-gate':

In this representation, the consumer is naïve, somewhat hapless and has been duped by the complexities of the agri-food industry … . What is required, then, the narrative goes, is enhanced awareness of our food chains, a reconnection to "local" and "national" foods and trusted sources, and an education that will help consumers make "better choices". (Abbots and Coles 2013: 544)

---

16   9 March 2014, https://twitter.com/ProfTimNoakes/status/442708225486782464.
17   11 April 2104, https://twitter.com/ProfTimNoakes/status/454704908613472256.
18   11 February 2014, https://twitter.com/ashman_65/status/433305780318904320.
19   16 April 2104, https://twitter.com/ProfTimNoakes/status/456501396963999745.
20   28 April 2014, https://twitter.com/OzParadoxdotcom/status/460728008794312704.

What these examples of Paleo/LCHF/Banting discourses and lifestyles do is to offer, through this 'enhanced awareness', a way to seize that control over personal choices. This is accomplished both through gaining more knowledge and, importantly, sharing that experience, which is where we see the richness of social media as Lomborg's 'communicative genre', rather than simply a technological development. So, as with Pollan's humanist tracts, these projects are at once personal and public: every LCHF success story contributes to the 'tipping point' that Noakes and others envisage happening:

> @ProfTimNoakes: #RealMealRevolution completes 10th consecutive week as top selling book in South Africa. Will South Africa be 1st country to "tip" to LCHF?

> @Gesundheith_SA: @ProfTimNoakes Congratulations to all you are a brave man. I am converted #LCHF and I will definitely spread this way of living.[21]

Yet where the sharing facility of social media arguably becomes problematic is when personal agendas are presumed to be appropriate for everyone, particularly when advocating a health behaviour not yet supported by conclusive evidence of being safe to follow in the long term. In other words, when sharing personal choices (via Twitter in this instance) *becomes* a mode of caring about other people's preferences, as illustrated by the following exchange involving, among others, this author:

> @sacrisis: @WOOLWORTHS_SA Get execs to read @ProfTimNoakes book & reduce low fat bull-shit products on your shelves & bring in more healthy full fat

> @Dr_Rousseau: @sacrisis In fact some people quite enjoy those "bullshit" low-fat products and don't need your dietary advice, thanks.

> @Ikhukhu: @Dr_Rousseau Well said. No need to turn individual dietary choices into a holy war.

> @Topcherry001pc: Woolies also sucked in by lo-fat dogma. They'll change as dictated by buying habits of customers[22]

Here again we see the theme of being 'duped', yet this time the 'victim' is Woolworths (a food and clothing retail chain), whose adherence to the 'lo-fat

---

21   27 April 214, https://twitter.com/ProfTimNoakes/status/460434362761093120.
22   30 March 2014, https://twitter.com/sacrisis/status/450184409258676224.

dogma' in turn makes ostensible victims of the consumers who evidently do not have the choice of 'good' full fat products when shopping.[23]

Indeed, if there is a prevailing sentiment in media discussions about food and public health, it is one of suspicion and distrust, with not infrequent gestures at conspiracy theories and ulterior motives.[24] This is the climate that accuses manufacturers of Girl Scout cookies of 'profiteering off an obvious public health problem' (Barclay 2014: np), and normalizes scepticism (if not outright cynicism) about, for example, whether a company like Coca-Cola can legitimately be involved in obesity research and interventions (Husten 2014). (The regularity of versions of the latter example prompted the Obesity Society to issue a position statement in March 2104 condemning ad hominem attacks on researchers with ties to 'suspicious' funding, stressing that 'funding source is not a sufficient basis upon which to discount otherwise sound scientific evidence', Obesity Society 2014).[25] Unsurprisingly, nurturing distrust in 'conventional' authorities routinely results in the manufacture of new sites of authority and expertise – in this case the maverick Professor considered brave enough to challenge existing 'dogma'. Once again, this is by no means exclusive to social media (the countercultural 70s could not have existed if this was the case), but the speed of progressions like this support Ritzer's notion of new technologies like these simply foregrounding and making more visible a historical 'means of prosumption'. Social media in this way can function not only as mechanisms of sharing and (s)caring, but also to unveil the construction (and sometimes disruption) of social structures governing the prescriptions of how and what to eat.

---

23   Part of the reasoning behind the LCHF eating plan is that fats have been unfairly maligned by nutritional guidelines, and also that low-fat products encourage the overconsumption of carbohydrates (often through added sugars), thought to be a key driver of obesity and diabetes.

24   See for example The Food Babe (foodbabe.com), a blog dedicated to investigating 'what's really in your food' by American blogger Vani Hari. In 2014, she infamously uncovered that the chain restaurant Subway used a chemical in their bread which is also found in yoga mats, and successfully campaigned for the company to change its bread recipe, despite there being no scientific evidence of any dangers to human health from ingesting said chemical (Novella 2014). At the time of writing, Hari had close to 700,000 fans on Facebook, and had most recently authored a blog post titled 'There Might Be Dead Animal Parts in your V8! & Homemade V8 Juice Recipe'.

25   As the author of a preliminary study of the effects of media exposure to contradictory nutrition messages concludes, one potential concern of this 'distrust' trope is that it could 'undermine the success of healthy eating campaigns and interventions. If people notice contradictory information about wine, fish, and other topics, and ultimately begin to doubt nutrition research and recommendations, then they might be less receptive to *subsequent* nutrition and non-nutrition related health campaign messages – perhaps even rejecting them altogether' (Nagler 2013).

#notyourgoodfatty

If embracing the LCHF lifestyle is one way to stage careful eating by seizing control out of the hands of 'experts' of one's food and body, a very different mode of caring is offered in the community of people who refuse to conform to one version of an 'ideal' weight. This is the ethos behind Fat Acceptance (FA)[26] and Health at Every Size (HAES) movements, which, as their names suggest, challenge what they see as the reductionist conflation of health with weight. Amanda Levitt, an 'Unapologetic Fat Lady' and host of the blog Fat Body Politics, outlines some of the key issues facing the community:

> The lack of diversity is a huge issue in the community and that even harms the reality of what it means to be a fat person in regards to health, because when everyone thinks that fat people are white and middle class they falsely believe we all have access to health behaviors. This places soul [sic] blame on individual fat people for performing health in a way our society deems acceptable … . People who demand we conform to an inaccessible performance of fatness, one that is based on proving health, are not actually interested in the humanity of fat people but in us performing for them and their comfort.

> Those demands also harm fat people in the community who don't perform fatness in a "socially acceptable" way due to numerous reasons but overwhelmingly you see that it has more to do with lack of access to health behaviors than just purely not caring. (Levitt 2014: np)

In keeping with this language of *performance*, it was Levitt who coined the hashtag #NotYourGoodFatty as a way to publicly – or at least on Twitter – challenge how fat people are perceived and treated. As she concludes: 'I'm not interested in performing fat positivity in a way that harms other fat people by letting outsiders know I am meeting their demands on my body. I want to challenge those demands' (ibid.).

Michelle Allison, who blogs under the moniker The Fat Nutritionist, and tweets as the @fatnutritionist, demonstrates:

> I'm not insulting myself when I call myself fat. Your assumption that I hate myself is pretty insulting though. #notyourgoodfatty

---

26   In the US, The National Association for the Advancement of Fat Acceptance was founded in 1969, and reportedly found 'new life' in the last decade or so thanks to FA blogs and other Internet-based activity (Honan 2009). For background on fat acceptance movement in the US, see for example Saguy and Riley (2005).

If you actually cared about fat people's health, you'd let them exist in the world in peace. Harassment is not helpful. #notyourgoodfatty

Judging someone as automatically less valuable due to a physical trait is bigotry. Congratulations, you're a bad person. #notyourgoodfatty

Appearance-based discrimination is wrong. Telling people they are disgusting "for their own good" is wrong. #notyourgoodfatty

Remember always, fat people: People are afraid of you because you have an awesome power – to destroy the hierarchy. #notyourgoodfatty[27]

In a follow-up post clarifying what is (and is not) meant by the hashtag, Allison explains further, emphasizing what she believes to be the limits on other people's authority to comment on and/or interfere with her size:

Random strangers on the street shouting abuse at fat people "for their own good"? No. Not acceptable. Doctors withholding effective treatment for certain health issues on the condition that fat people engage in a risky, non-evidence-based treatment (dieting)? No. Not acceptable, and not health-promoting. Well-meaning but ignorant, or even frankly abusive, family members or friends tossing off health advice to adults who have not solicited it? No. Not acceptable. (Allison 2014: np)

Allison's follow-up post was inspired by the (somewhat predictable) misuse of the hashtag, as if to give credence to the kind of abuse it was meant to confront. Yet even here, the sense of a caring – and cared for – community appears to trump the naysayers, putting agency and authority squarely in the hands of the #notgoodfatties:

@karenczmills: Trolls don't bother me. You can't take this positive activism experience from me. I will not give you that power. #notyourgoodfatty[28]

@Artists_Ali: There should be a new fatty hashtag since #notyourgoodfatty is overrun w/ Reddit trolls.

---

27   These tweets (from 4th-5th April 2014) were 'Storified' (Storify being another social media application designed to collect media and 'make the web tell a story', https://storify.com), and can be viewed collectively at https://storify.com/marxroadrunner/fatnutritionist-being-amazing-on-the-notyourgoodfa.
28   15 April 2014, https://twitter.com/karenczmills/status/455940008193425408.

@Ravenverde: @Artists_Ali I've blocked them all, so for me, #notyourgoodfatty is full of strong fatties and their supporters.[29]

To bring the discussion back to the – often false – dichotomies between what is 'good' and 'bad' when it comes to eating behaviours, Shaunta Grimes (HAES advocate, and member of FA web-based collective Fierce Freethinking Fatties) points out that:

> Interestingly, the opposite of a Good Fatty isn't a Bad Fatty … . [T]he opposite of a Good Fatty is a fat person who does not need to justify or apologize for their existence or for the existence of fat people in the world. If we eat donuts, we're still valuable. If we don't exercise, we're still valuable. Even if we're not healthy, we're still valuable. The opposite of a Good Fatty is a fat rebel who believes in autonomy and that a person's health is a personal concern and not up for public debate. (Grimes 2014: np)

As we have seen with the example of the LCHF lifestyle, creating communities of both care and dissent, such as those inhabited by #notyourgoodfattys, is not limited to social media, but these digital tools certainly do facilitate the rapid expansion of, and by extension support for, such groups. Perhaps a more noteworthy feature of the social mediascape is how the same mechanisms that allow for rapid expansion (as in the case of such open, rather than closed, or subscription-only groups) disallows privacy. In short, if you want to trend on Twitter, you are of necessity open to public scrutiny, and thereby also vulnerable to abuse by 'trolls'. And while the examples above demonstrate an asserted robustness in the face of such abuse, the apparatuses which conduce to confirmation bias are no less at play here: by blocking all the 'Reddit trolls', this particular user also succeeds in using Twitter to create an echo chamber of virtual support, where dissenting views are essentially prohibited and this particular configuration of authority remains inviolable. While this perhaps succeeds in creating a safe and unthreatening virtual space, it is also a space which translates very poorly to the 'real world' where discrimination continues for the most part unabated (Abrams 2012; Berlant 2007; Christian 2007; Slocum et al. 2011).

As Grimes makes clear in her description of the opposite of a 'Good Fatty', the (self-formulated) question here is not so much one of health, as it is of value, privacy and the authority both to care and to share. Yet, the description of 'autonomy' as being ultimately extrinsic to public life and debate is also at odds with the logic of #notyourgoodfatty, which is about proclaiming that autonomy on a public platform. It is about asking for attention from and then rejecting any accountability to that public. This is not to argue against the perfectly reasonable premise that someone is of value even if they are not healthy, but there is also a certain disingenuity underlying the idea that personal choices (should) have no public ramifications.

---

29 22 April, https://twitter.com/Artists_Ali/status/458581804640124929.

The lines are sometimes subtle, but often less so, between using tools like social media to exhibit, 'perform', or 'produse' behaviours that contribute to disabling rather than enabling someone. As Dr. David Katz (Director of the Yale University Prevention Research Centre) summarized a recently published study examining the correlations between fatness and fitness that challenge the idea of 'healthy obesity' thanks to the increase in coronary calcification with excess weight, the results generated:

> a potentially important message that argues back against the "ok at any size movement". Size may be ok, but coronary disease is not. If we have to control our body fat to prevent calcified plaque in our coronary arteries, that is not a body image issue; it's a matter of potentially life and death significance. (Katz 2014: np)[30]

Matters of life and death are rarely entirely private matters, and especially not when they are rehearsed on publicly accessible social media networks.

On Whose Authority?

Underpinning many of these debates and online performances of ideological positions about what constitutes careful eating is the question of why anyone should care about what others eat, and indeed who has the right to intervene – or interfere, as I have called an unwarranted intervention elsewhere (Rousseau 2012a) – in others' choices. The examples surveyed so far illustrate a variety of motives, from nurturing our humanity through caring for the planet in the case of cultured beef, to seizing control from the 'traditional' experts through an LCHF lifestyle, to giving a proverbial finger to the body police by refusing to be a #goodfatty. Diverse as the end results of each of these positions may be, they all take part in a contemporary 'democratization' of knowledge and expertise, which is fuelled in significant part by the mechanics of the web and social media that facilitate the very active use (and re-use, and sometimes abuse, for the sake of sensation and/or fear-mongering) of an exponentially expanding databank of information. It is quite possibly this relatively recent opening up of conversations about what were previously specialized fields – here, genetic engineering, nutrition, public health – which both destabilizes public perception in traditional expertise, and also generates expectations in finding (or creating) authority from non-conventional sites.[31]

---

30   See also Sainsbury and Hay (2014), who argue for an 'urgent rethink of the "health at every size" concept'.

31   While lay individuals have arguably had and shared opinions on topics beyond their expertise well before the advent of social media, today's digital climate is unique in that it has enabled and normalized a more eclectic pool of interlocutors in any given

The chef industry is a case in point, as Anthony Bourdain points out in an interview with (chef and food writer) Michael Ruhlman:

> Ruhlman: When you choose to be a chef, what are your obligations, if any?

> Bourdain: Increasingly there are obligations. In my generation I don't think there were, we didn't think about any obligation. We were in the pleasure business, that was it. Your only obligation was to give your customers a good time at a price point they found reasonable. And you didn't care where the tomato came from as long as it was a pleasure-giving tomato. That dynamic has changed. Chefs think about that stuff now. Because the issues are raised and discussed within the community. Because chefs are either being pushed to be citizens of the world or are just naturally thinking about these things from the get-go. These were not issues we thought about back then. (Ruhlman 2014: np)

The changing 'dynamic' that Bourdain refers to here is at least in part driven by digital advances which mean that it has become increasingly difficult to continue to, for example, not *publicly* care about where a tomato comes from if all your peers do.[32] Although the provenance of a tomato is an admittedly frivolous example, it speaks to the much broader paradigm of care that describes an attitude to the world, and to others. And this is a conversation that goes beyond the professional chef community to be alive and well on social media platforms, where chefs and other food personalities are often scrutinized for behaviours not even related to food, and where crowds can turn harsh if they do not like what they see.[33]

Jamie Oliver is one chef who seems particularly adept at annoying people, but the example of whom is particularly instructive when it comes to the often contradictory concerns around the expectations, responsibilities and entitlements relating to public conversations about how we ought to eat. Oliver's career to-date exemplifies the contemporary expansion of the expertise of a chef, as in a professional who is trained to cook for other people. In addition to the environmental

---

conversation. So it is not unusual to see scientists in public conversations with non-scientists on Twitter. Closer to intellectual (as opposed to scientific) pursuits related to food and eating is the example of restaurant reviewing, where the professional critic is now in increasing competition with amateur bloggers, and crowd-sourced review sites like Yelp for public attention.

32   One of the first web-based scandals in the professional cooking world was when examples of culinary plagiarism were revealed by which a restaurant in Sydney had reproduced without credit dishes from well-known American restaurants Alinea and WD-50. The similarities were noted thanks to pictures of the dishes being posted on the restaurant website.

33   For example when television cook Ina Garten, also known as the 'Barefoot Contessa', was maligned for supposedly refusing the wish – via the *Make-A-Wish Foundation* – of a young fan and cancer patient. For this and other examples, see Rousseau (2012b).

matters that inform Bourdain's version of how to be a 'good citizen', these include in Oliver's case issues related to public health and nutrition, particularly in the context of childhood obesity (Rousseau 2102a). When promoting his then-latest venture *Jamie's Money Saving Meals* in 2013, Oliver made reference to how people on limited budgets eat in Mediterranean countries, with the perceived insinuation that they managed this 'better' than their British counterparts:

> I meet people who say, 'You don't understand what it's like'. I just want to hug them and teleport them to the Sicilian street cleaner who has 25 mussels, 10 cherry tomatoes, and a packet of spaghetti for 60 pence, and knocks out the most amazing pasta. You go to Italy or Spain and they eat well on not much money. We've missed out on that in Britain, somehow. (quoted in Deans 2013: np)

Oliver's remarks generated a variety of reactions that do well to summarize the controversies underlying the very idea of a generalized philosophy of how to (and who can) perform care. One writer opined that although he believes that Oliver's 'heart is in the right place', he 'needs to stop publishing books, the last one of which was judged one of the unhealthiest on the market, while internally tutting at the deplorable lack of quinoa in "poor communities"' (Andreou 2013: np). Another criticized Oliver for furthering a myth of 'authentic peasant food', which not only ('wrongly', it is implied) upholds an extremely lucrative cookbook, restaurant chain and food television empire in the UK and the US, but also perpetuates a classist notion of the 'deserving poor', as opposed to the British poor whose habits Oliver laments (McCormack 2013).

In a defence (of sorts) was the argument that while Oliver might not be an expert in the field of either nutrition or poverty, his experience grants him more authority than most:

> It's pretty bloody rich that one might look at a cookery expert like Oliver – who became fixated some years back on giving cookery classes to the poor, teaching impoverished kids what vegetable [sic] looks like, negotiating with dinner ladies about budgets, fighting with local government and the actual prime minister on the matter of how to break the vicious circle which leads to child existing on chips and cheese – and shout back at him, 'Well what do you know about how poor people feed their children?' The fact is: probably much more than you. (Dent 2013: np)

In a post entitled 'Jamie Oliver Should Stop Trying to Teach Poor People How to Eat', finally, an American writer agrees with the previously cited suggestion that the chef is 'entitled' to his opinions, but concludes that 'he's not entitled to the position of culinary hero for a population he disdains' (Anderson 2013: np). A few weeks after the incident, Oliver himself acknowledged the indignation that he had caused, but claimed to be undeterred: 'If I don't say these things, no one else fucking will. The government doesn't like to say stuff like that because they're chasing votes. I'm in the slight luxury of not being able to get myself fired. The public are my first boss' (quoted in Lewis 2013: np).

These pronouncements speak to an intriguing interplay of care and disdain that frame not only this isolated example (on both the sides of Oliver and of his critics), but publicly staged conversations about 'proper' eating in general. While Oliver claims to be motivated by care for those he intends to help, some of his critics disallow that possibility because of his wealth, suggesting instead the more cynical motive of capitalizing on a group whom he actively dislikes. But besides this being a classic example of a 'damned if he does, damned if he doesn't', more notable in the context of the main concerns of this chapter is the frequency with which normative language is marshalled to address situations which are clearly more complex and nuanced than such prescriptions allow. 'Should' a celebrity chef be involved in teaching poor people how to eat? Not according to his job description, no. But that does not prohibit him from attempting to do so, any more than it should prevent an accountant from volunteering at a soup kitchen – *if* such involvements are welcomed by the their supposed beneficiaries. 'Should' an overweight person be pressured into losing weight to conform to an 'acceptable' BMI? Not if they do not put themselves or others at risk, or represent an undue burden on public healthcare costs, in which case it would be reasonable to extract higher premiums (as with smokers, who pay more for the freedom to put themselves at risk). 'Should' we eschew lab-grown, or genetically modified, foods in favour of those that are local, organic, unsullied by Big Food and by the compromised ethics of traditional 'experts'? Well, clearly yes. And clearly no.

Conclusion

It should hopefully be clear that each of the responses to the questions above are themselves loaded, and could be complicated much further in trying to ascertain who has the right to decide what is 'best' (what if, for example, poor people do *not* welcome Jamie Oliver's involvement? Would a government intervention be more appropriate? Is *any* intervention appropriate? And so on). It should hopefully also be evident that there is some dimension of all the issues discussed in this chapter which have little to do with social media, and which would likely continue to be divisive without these digital facilities.

But digital technologies like social media have long ceased to be an optional extra for purely recreational purposes. While they certainly continue to provide that function, the merely 'social' part of the technology now exists in addition to the many more consequential activities we see unfolding on these platforms, among them debates and nascent movements – some indeed worthy of the name crusades – related to 'good' and 'proper' eating. In this way Stine Lomborg is absolutely correct in calling the very term social media 'nonsense', but not because 'it presumes that other communication media are not social' (Lomborg

2011: 56). Rather, it is a nonsense term because of how little of the activity that the technology facilitates is accurately described by the term 'social'.

There can be no doubting the net positives afforded by the digital age, including unprecedented access to information, and the formation and maintenance of countless virtual communities. But at least some of that social media activity, as the examples in this chapter collectively demonstrate, conduce to less productive results like confirmation bias and the generation of false dichotomies that this concluding exchange from Noakes' timeline both satirizes and illustrates:

> @PrimalPerks: Interesting how either people love disussing [sic] @ ProfTimNoakes diet or they consider his name a swear word! Reckon those are the carb addicts.

> @ProfTimNoakes: @PrimalPerks Even for scientists, nutrition is a religion. So I am either the Patron Saint or the excommunicated Heretic. No in-between.[34]

It is tempting to speculate, as others have done,[35] about whether it is the technology itself that is to blame. But as psychologists Daniel Kahneman and Amos Tversky (1974) pointed out several decades ago already, human beings excelled at cognitive biases and logical fallacies long before any digital age. What social media do instead is afford us is the opportunity to observe social hierarchies at work, which includes the twin dynamics of consent and resistance as new voices and authorities make themselves heard.

So it is perhaps also to be expected that while the digital tools we have available to us can certainly enhance our lives, they can – and clearly do – also exacerbate the things we already do badly, like impatiently preferring the simplistic over the nuanced. Once again, this is not to blame technology, but rather to acknowledge its facilitating role in what one social scientist describes as a 'hunger for fast, definitive answers' (quoted in Adler 2013: np) in which everyone, lay and professional alike, is complicit. Here we see one of the consequences of 'mediated mobilism', whereby social media at once facilitate and indeed compel the simultaneous consumption and production of information. As active prosumers, we inhabit a more democratic, and therefore empowering, knowledge landscape. But as we have seen with the examples in this chapter, it is also a space in which hierarchies of authority and expertise can become exposed and disrupted in ways that are not uniformly constructive. Combined with the notion that 'all that happens must be known' (the very art-imitates-life motto of a fictional social media company in David Eggers 2014 novel *The Circle*), these vagaries of mobility could, in the end,

---

34   4 May 2014, https://twitter.com/ProfTimNoakes/status/463029455850856449.

35   For example Nicholas Carr, who famously asked if 'Google is making us stupid' in an essay for *The Atlantic* which was later developed into the book *The Shallows: What the Internet is Doing to Our Brains* (Carr 2010).

function most successfully at generating a recipe for *not* thinking very carefully about how to eat.

References

Abbots, E-J. and Coles, B. 2013. Horsemeat-gate: The discursive production of a neoliberal food scandal. *Food, Culture and Society*, 16(4), 535-50.

Abrams, L. 2012. Think of the (fat) children: Minnesota's "better example" anti-obesity campaign. *The Atlantic*, 24 September [online]. Available at: http://www.theatlantic.com/health/archive/2012/09/think-of-the-fat-children-minnesotas-better-example-anti-obesity-campaign/262674 [accessed: 24 September 2012].

Adler, J. 2014. The reformation: Can social scientists save themselves? *Pacific Standard*, 28 April [online]. Available at: http://www.psmag.com/navigation/health-and-behavior/can-social-scientists-save-themselves-human-behavior-78858 [accessed: 28 April 2014].

Allison, M. 2014. What I'm saying, and what I'm not saying. *The Fat Nutritionist*, 7 April 2014 [online]. Available at: http://www.fatnutritionist.com/index.php/what-im-saying-and-what-im-not-saying [accessed: 10 April 2014].

Anderson, L.V. 2013. Jamie Oliver should stop trying to teach poor people how to eat. *Slate*, 30 August [online]. Available at: http://www.slate.com/blogs/browbeat/2013/08/30/jamie_oliver_s_classism_the_naked_chef_is_not_the_right_person_to_teach.html [accessed: 5 September 2013].

Andreou, A. 2013. Jamie Oliver, you haven't tasted real poverty. Cut out the tutting. *The Guardian*, 27 August [online]. Available at: http://www.theguardian.com/commentisfree/2013/aug/27/jamie-oliver-poverty-ready-meals-tv [accessed: 10 September 2013].

AP. 2009. Nobel prize winner Norman Borlaug dies at 95. *Associated Press*, 13 September [online]. Available at: http://www.nbcnews.com/id/32821828/ns/us_news-environment/t/nobel-prize-winner-norman-borlaug-dies/#.U1zdHPmSxoQ [accessed: 2 July 2013].

Baggini, J. 2013. The vegan carnivore? *Aeon Magazine*, 3 September [online]. Available at: http://aeon.co/magazine/nature-and-cosmos/in-vitro-meat-demands-a-whole-new-food-ethics [accessed: 16 January 2014].

Barclay, E. 2014. Do girl scout cookies still make the world a better Place? *NPR*, 1 April [online]. Available at: http://www.npr.org/blogs/thesalt/2014/04/01/295748000/do-girl-scout-cookies-still-make-the-world-a-better-place [accessed: 3 April 2014].

Berlant, L. 2007. Slow death (sovereignty, obesity, lateral agency). *Critical Inquiry*, 33(4), 754-80.

Brewster, S. 2013. Testers claim lab-grown burger backed by Sergey Brin had nice texture, bland flavor. *Gigaom*, 5 August [online]. Available at: http://gigaom.com/2013/08/05/testers-claim-lab-grown-burger-backed-by-sergey-brin-had-nice-texture-bland-flavor [accessed: 7 August 2014].

Bruns, A. 2008. *Blogs, Wikipedia, Second Life, and Beyond: From Production to Produsage.* New York: Peter Lang.

Campos, P., Saguy, A., Ernsberger, P., Oliver, E. and Gaesser, G. 2006. The epidemiology of overweight and obesity: Public health crisis or moral panic? *International Journal of Epidemiology*, 35(1), 55-60.

Carr, N. 2010. *The Shallows: What the Internet is Doing to Our Brains.* New York and London: Norton & Company.

Carruth, A. 2013. Michael Pollan's dilemma. *Public Books*, 1 November [online]. Available at: http://www.publicbooks.org/nonfiction/michael-pollans-dilemma [accessed: 7 December 2013].

Christian, N. 2007. Shame game 'losing' war on obesity. *The Scotsman*, 21 July [online]. Available at: http://news.scotsman.com/latestnews/Shame-game-losing-war-on.3309001.jp [accessed: 5 August 2010].

Connor, S. 2014. Former Greenpeace leading light condemns them for opposing GM 'golden rice' crop that could save two million children from starvation per year. *The Independent*, 30 January [online]. Available at: http://www.independent. co.uk/news/science/former-greenpeace-leading-light-condemns-them-for-opposing-gm-golden-rice-crop-that-could-save-two-million-children-from-starvation-per-year-9097170.html [accessed: 10 February 2014].

Danovich, T. 2014. Where did the food movement go wrong? *Food Politic*, 20 March [online]. Available at: http://www.foodpolitic.com/where-did-the-food-movement-go-wrong [accessed: 16 April 2014].

Deans, J. 2013. Jamie Oliver bemoans chips, cheese and giant TVs of modern-day poverty. *The Guardian*, 27 August [online]. Available at: http://www. theguardian.com/lifeandstyle/2013/aug/27/jamie-oliver-chips-cheese-modern-day-poverty [accessed: 5 September 2013].

Dent, G. 2013. Stop slagging off Jamie Oliver. He's earned the right to these opinions. *The Independent*, 28 August [online]. Available at: http://www.independent. co.uk/voices/comment/stop-slagging-off-jamie-oliver-hes-earned-the-right-to-these-opinions-8788228.html [accessed: 10 September 2013].

Eggers, D. 2014. *The Circle.* New York: Knopf.

Gard, M. and Wright, J. 2005. *The Obesity Epidemic: Science, Morality, and Ideology.* London: Routledge.

Grimes, S. 2014. Guest pots: I am no one's good fatty. *Skepchick*, 21 April [online]. Available at: http://skepchick.org/2014/04/guest-post-i-am-no-ones-good-fatty [accessed: 24 April 2014].

Haidt, J. 2001. The emotional dog and its rational tail: A social intuitionist approach to moral judgment. *Psychological Review*, 108(4), 814-34.

Harmon, A. 2013. Golden rice: Lifesaver? *New York Times*, 24 August [online]. http://www.nytimes.com/2013/08/25/sunday-review/golden-rice-lifesaver. html [accessed: 2 February 2014].

Hartmann, M. 2013. From domestication to mediated mobilism. *Mobile Media & Communication*, 1(1), 42-9.

Honan, E. 2009. Obesity becoming U.S. civil rights issue for some. *Reuters*, 27 April [online]. Available at: http://www.reuters.com/article/2009/04/28/us-obesity-acceptance-idUSTRE53R00Z20090428 [accessed: 20 October 2010].

Humes, L., Runquist, C. and Weldon, K. 2014. In vitro meat: A bunch of bologna? *The Mac Weekly*, 18 April [online]. Available at: http://themacweekly.com/2014/04/in-vitro-meat-a-bunch-of-bologna [accessed: 18 April 2014].

Husten, Larry. 2014. What role should Coca-Cola play in obesity research? *Forbes*, 27 April [online]. http://www.forbes.com/sites/larryhusten/2014/04/27/what-role-should-coca-cola-play-in-obesity-research/2 [accessed: 27 April 2014].

Kahneman, D. and Tversky, A. 1974. Judgments under uncertainty: Heuristics and biases. *Science*, 185(4157), 1124-31.

Kandil, C.Y. 2013. Michael Pollan: High priest of American food. *Moment*, July-August [online]. Available at: http://www.momentmag.com/michael-pollan-high-priest-of-american-food [accessed: 10 November 2013].

Katz, D. 2014. Fatness and our arterial fitness. *LinkedIn*, 2 May [online]. Available at: https://www.linkedin.com/today/post/article/20140502120252-23027997-fatness-and-our-arterial-fitness [accessed: 2 May 2014].

LeBesco, K. 2010. Fat panic and the new morality, in *Against Health: How Health Became the New Morality*, edited by J.M. Metzl and A. Kirkland. New York and London: New York University Press, 72-82.

Levitt, A. 2014. #NotYourGoodFatty – The performing fatty. *Fat Body Politics*, 4 April [online]. Available at: http://fatbodypolitics.com/2014/04/04/notyourgoodfatty-and-the-performing-fatty [accessed: 6 April 2014].

Lewis, T. 2013. Jamie Oliver: 'I cause a storm every time I open my mouth'. *The Observer*, 19 October [online]. Available at: http://www.theguardian.com/lifeandstyle/2013/oct/19/jamie-oliver-i-cause-a-storm [accessed: 2 December 2013].

Lomborg, S. 2011. Social media as communicative genres. *MedieKultur*, 27(51), 55-71.

Mattick, A. and Allenby, B. 2014. The future of meat. *Issues in Science and Technology*, 5 February [online]. Available at: http://issues.org/30-1/carolyn [accessed: 10 March 2014].

McCormack, R. 2013. Dear Jamie Oliver, poverty isn't picturesque by the Mediterranean either. *New Statesman*, 27 August [online]. Available at: http://www.newstatesman.com/food-and-drink/2013/08/dear-jamie-oliver-poverty-isnt-picturesque-mediterranean-either [accessed: 10 September 2103].

Nagler, R. 2013. Adverse outcomes associated with media exposure to contradictory nutrition messages. *Journal of Health Communication: International Perspectives*, 19(1), 24-40.

Novella, S. 2014. Eating yoga mats. *Neurologica*, 14 February [online]. Available at: http://theness.com/neurologicablog/index.php/eating-yoga-mats [accessed: 15 February 2014].

Obesity Society 2014. Science-industry collaborations can support obesity science, public health. *Obesity Society: Research. Education. Action*, 24 March [online]. Available at: http://www.obesity.org/news-center/science-industry-collaborations-can-support-obesity-science-public-health.htm [accessed: 4 April 2014].

Pariser, E. 2011. Beware online "filter bubbles". *TED*, 3 May [online]. Available at: http://www.thefilterbubble.com/ted-talk [accessed: 2 March 2014].

Ritzer, G. 2014. Prosumption: Evolution, revolution, or eternal return of the same? *Journal of Consumer Culture*, 14(1), 3-24.

Ritzer, G. and Jurgenson, N. 2010. Production, consumption, presumption: The nature of capitalism in the age of the digital 'prosumer'. *Journal of Consumer Culture*, 10(1), 13-36.

Ritzer, G., Dean, P. and Jurgenson, N. 2012. The coming of age of the prosumer. *American Behavioral Scientist*, 56(4), 379-98.

Rousseau, S. 2012a. *Food Media: Celebrity Chefs and the Politics of Everyday Interference*. Oxford: Berg.

Rousseau, S. 2012b. *Food and Social Media: You Are What You Tweet*. Lanham: Altamira.

Ruhlman, M. 2014. Anthony Bourdain on today's chefs. *Ruhlman*, 26 February [online]. Available at: http://ruhlman.com/2014/02/anthony-bourdain-on-todays-chefs [accessed: 10 March 2014].

Saguy, A.C. and Riley, K.W. 2005. Weighing both sides: Morality, mortality, and framing contests over obesity. *Journal of Health Politics, Policy and Law*, 30, 869-923.

Sainsbury, A. and Hay, P. 2014. Call for an urgent rethink of the 'health at every size' concept. *Journal of Eating Disorders*, 2(8), available at http://www.ncbi.nlm.nih.gov/pmc/articles/PMC3995323/pdf/2050-2974-2-8.pdf [accessed: 24 October 2014].

Slocum, R., Shannon, J., Cadieux, K.V. and Beckman, M. 2011. 'Properly, with love, from scratch': Jamie Oliver's food revolution. *Radical History Review*, 110 (Spring), 178-91.

Strauss, E. 2012. The terrible tragedy of the healthy eater. *Northwest Edible* Life, 1 August [online]. Available at: http://www.nwedible.com/2012/08/tragedy-healthy-eater.html [accessed: 2 February 2014].

Taubes, G. 2002. What if it's all been a big fat lie? *New York Times* [online]. Available at: http://www.nytimes.com/2002/07/07/magazine/what-if-it-s-all-been-a-big-fat-lie.html [accessed: 7 July 2012].

Taubes, G. 2007. *The Diet Delusion*. London: Vermillion.

Teicholz, N. 2014. *The Big Fat Surprise: Why Butter, Meat and Cheese Belong in a Healthy Diet*. New York and London: Simon and Schuster.

Zuckerman, E. 2008. Homophily, serendipity, xenophilia. *My Heart's in Accra*, 25 April [online]. Available at: http://www.ethanzuckerman.com/blog/2008/04/25/homophily-serendipity-xenophilia [accessed: 5 July 2102].

Zuk, M. 2013. *Paleofantasy: What Evolution Really Tells Us About Sex, Diet, and How We Live*. New York: W.W. Norton & Company.

Chapter 3

Caring about Careless Eating: Class Politics, Governance and the Production of Otherness in Highland Ecuador

Emma-Jayne Abbots

Introduction

This chapter explores the ways in which care is politically deployed in the Southern Ecuadorian Andes. Specifically, I consider how particular groups mobilize care in myriad ways to critique, interfere and govern Other people's eating by appealing beyond the health of the eaters' individual bodies to that of the broader social body. Put simply, I elucidate how particular social groups, in this context the local Cuencano population and the migrant-peasantry, are subjected to visions of 'good food' perpetuated by other social groups structurally positioned above them in the social order – privileged migrants and the governing class. As such, I interrogate what constitutes 'careful eating' and examine how subjective notions of care-full (Miele and Evans 2010) and care-less food work to establish social distance and produce otherness. My aim in this chapter is, therefore, to demonstrate how discourses of good food and proper eating that are ostensibly premised on caring-for the corporeal bodies of Others and appear benign are, instead, politically motivated and centred on caring-about wider social issues.

The ethnography on which I draw is set in the greater Cuenca region of the Southern Ecuadorian Andes. Colloquially known as 'the Athens of Ecuador', the region is renowned for its pre-Inca ruins, Spanish colonial architecture and a rich tradition in literature and the arts. It is also arguably the whitest and most conservative areas of Ecuador and a deeply entrenched class hierarchy, which intersects with ethnicity, kinship and ideas of 'cultured' (read white urban) behaviour, continues to permeate every facet of social and cultural life. Outside of Cuenca city – a UNESCO world heritage site – the landscape contains a number of small rural and semi-rural communities, which have historically relied on small and medium scale agriculture as their primary economic strategy. This heritage is valued, celebrated and marketed, and made materially manifest in the form of the *Chola Cuencana* – a mixed-race, female folkloric figure that straddles both the country and the city (see Abbots 2014a; Weismantel 2001, 2003). However, the economy of these communities has been transformed in recent years as the area has witnessed extensive and sustained outward migration to the USA and Europe following national economic crisis and the collapse of the rural economy in the late 1990s. The resultant remittance incomes have resulted in the emergence of a newly-wealthy migrant-peasant class, who are orientated towards being 'modern' and socially mobile (Abbots 2014a). More recently, the region has also received a number of more privileged migrants, primarily from North America, who are seeking a lifestyle change and in 2009 Cuenca was named 'The World's Best Retirement Haven' by *International Living* magazine (International Living 2010). This group, while small in number, are significantly shaping the local foodscape and engage readily with discourses of good food.

Throughout this chapter I draw on my fieldwork amongst this group of privileged migrants, as well as my research among the governing upper and middle classes (hereafter governing classes), who are primarily based in the city but also commonly have economic and social ties to, and actively govern, the *campo* (countryside) and *campesinos* (peasantry). Consequently, I also discuss those who have more humble economic origins and continue to reside in the *campo*, with whom I have lived with and conducted long-term extensive fieldwork primarily in the form of participant observation, group discussions and unstructured interviews. I prefer to refer to this group as the migrant-peasantry rather than the more commonly used *campesino*. This is because, while this social group are the longstanding local residents of the *campo* and define themselves as such, the international outward migration of their kin and the receipt of remittance incomes is now their household's primary economic strategy and they consciously reject small scale agricultural production and the social baggage which accompanies being *campesino*. Defining this group then as the migrant-peasantry best reflects their historical social and economic background as members of 'the peasantry' while also allowing for their current aspirations and economic practices, as well as the cultural expectations that are laid upon them by those 'higher' in the social order.

Whilst recognizing that individual subjectivities are multi-faceted (Ong 1999) and class categories are, in lived realities, more mutable and complex than academic analysis can fully account – as well as being mindful of the ways migration can destablilize class orders (Abbots 2012a) – clear class distinctions and tensions emerge between the groups I discuss below. Untangling the relationships between these socially different groups can, therefore, provide insights into the ways in which everyday food practices play a major role in the constitution and enactment of these class dynamics. I have addressed this theme previously (Abbots 2011, 2013, 2014b) and in this chapter I look to extend my earlier analysis of, and bring a fresh perspective to, the political entanglements between eating and class by viewing them through the rubric of care. This chapter thereby takes the stance that care is not politically benign but is instead a biopolitical instrument through which individual bodies can be regulated and governed. As such, it draws inspiration from a body of literature that demonstrates how caring is entangled with moral values (Barnes 2012) and enables the bodies of both carer and cared-for to be relationally co-produced (Mol 2010). Moreover, it plays with the notion that 'to care' is both a feeling (to care-about) and a practice (to care-for) (Ungerson 1983; Tronto 1993), and looks to build upon this multi-layered conceptualization of care by examining that ways that caring-for (Others) can obfuscate cares-about broader social issues. The slippery nature of care – and how this enables it to be deployed within class relations – is thus brought to the fore. In addition, my discussion implicates Foucauldian questions of governance (Foucault 1978), as I interrogate the ways in which privileged migrants and the governing classes construct (perceived) absences of care in the local Cuencano population and the migrant-peasantry as a problem that requires intervention. I consequently indicate how the bodies of some social groups are governed – or more accurately attempted to be governed – by an Other and elucidate how practices that seem to be premised on intimacies, closeness and concern are, instead, centred on the enactment and potential contestation of governmental power.

Privileged Migrants: Caring-about Local(s) Eating

> They don't know what they're doing: they're eating all this junk food and just don't realise what they're doing to their bodies – how bad it is for them. And the waste as well: the amount of rubbish that gets produced and just gets thrown all over the landscape – this beautiful landscape! It's being ruined.

The above was spoken by Angela, one of my research participants who had recently migrated to Ecuador from the USA, during a focus group discussion with a number of privileged migrants[1] on their eating preferences and practices. I use it as a springboard for this chapter as it not only indicates the ways in which this group voice their concerns about Other people's eating, but also suggests how multiple cares for healthy bodies and environments, and cares about the effects of the industrial food system, are entangled and crystallized under the rubric of careful eating. Privileged migrants, who predominantly originate from the USA but also come from Australasia and Europe, are moving to the greater Cuenca region in numbers significant enough to be socially visible and economically impactful. This group's motivations for making what, for many, is a socially, culturally and economically drastic move revolves around the desire for a more 'simple life' and 'simple food' (Abbots 2013: 121). Simple food meaning, in their words, concomitantly 'local', 'organic' and 'traditional, as well as preferably purchased 'directly off the people who grew it' such as 'the peasant women with the baskets and the wheelbarrows of fruit'. However, during the course of

---

1   These individuals are more commonly defined, and at times define themselves, as expatriates or expats. Drawing on Fechter (2007), I prefer to use the term 'privileged migrants' in acknowledgement that 'expatriate' is not a politically benign category.

our individual and group interviews about their own food practices, it was not uncommon for my participants to start talking, like Angela, about how and what Cuencanos, particularly those from the lower rungs of society, eat.

Returning to that focus group, Tammy picked up the conversational thread, agreeing with Angela's views and lamenting the perceived lack of fresh fruit and vegetables in the local population's diet and a heavy reliance on refined carbohydrates, stating; 'they have all these amazing fruit and veg here – it's so cheap and there is such a range, but they just don't eat them'. The two women ruminated on the health consequences of this diet, with Angela asking, 'I heard that stomach cancer is on the rise here, why do you think that is'? Cynthia offered an answer: 'they're a different build than us – short and stocky – so maybe they can eat differently'. 'But they eat so much more', Bryan interjected, '*mote* [a white corn] is so filling, I can only eat a small amount and I'm full, but they can eat loads of it'. The conversation turned towards what was generally understood as a Cuencano propensity for sugary sweet foods, and my participants highlighted the sweet treats associated with fiestas, as well as the large quantities of soft drinks consumed, with Bryan exclaiming 'and those bottles aren't small; 3 litres'! In turn, his wife Carol was concerned about the health of Cuencano children, and drew my attention to the 'food that is sold in the streets outside of schools – *salchipapas* [mini-hot dog sausages and chips] and fried foods and that foamy sweet ice-cream', which she stated was 'damaging to their health, right from the start – it's irresponsible'.

These understandings of Cuencano eating practices are arguably based more on preconceptions and casual observations, including that of body size and waistlines, rather than intimate acquaintance with the local population and they are, in many ways, self-(re)producing. Moreover, neither are they unexpected given my participants' views on the food industry more generally, and the fast-food sector specifically. All studiously avoided the two global chains most prevalent in Cuenca, Burger King and Kentucky Fried Chicken, and the popularity of these chains amongst Cuencanos was a cause of great despair, with Lois exclaiming, 'why are they eating this stuff when they have all this wonderful fresh produce?' Even the very presence of such chains was the cause of much disappointment and disdain, as privileged migrants came to the realization that 'they couldn't escape' such restaurants and the dynamics of globalization. The global chains and their products were consequently held up as markers of all they deemed wrong with the food system and were regarded as antithetical to the 'simple foods' and values upon which privileged migrants are trying to base their new lifestyles. Enmeshed within this discourse is the notion that the local population are not aware of the 'dangers' of eating 'bad' foods from global chains and, if they were, they would cease to do so. This is because, as Donna told me 'it's all new to them, it's still a novelty'. And, as Xenia surmised, 'well, they're [Cuencanos] just not as far along as us in realizing the dangers of *those* foods' (my emphasis). 'Those foods' meaning those that are regarded – within the polarized framework held by privileged migrants – as diametrically opposed to local, organic, simple and traditional. As such, the dangers are not limited to the effects on individual bodies, but also to the manner in which 'they erode the sites of simple food production, displace the local, and supplant tradition' (Abbots 2013: 125). Thus we start to see how caring-for the health of Cuencano bodies is shaped by and shrouds value-laden cares-about the contemporary food system. I develop this point below but first I want to attend to Xenia's contention that Cuencanos 'are just not as far along as us'. This statement, I suggest, warrants some unpacking in that it produces social distance between privileged migrants and Cuencanos, as well as drawing attention to the latter's absence of care.

'Just Not as Far Along': Experience, Knowledge and the Absence of Care

In stating that Cuencanos are not 'as far along' as privileged migrants, Xenia draws attention to her social group's greater awareness – and cares about – 'those foods' and their seemingly inherent risks. In contrast, Cuencanos are discursively constructed as lacking awareness and consequently, care. Because if they did have such knowledge and previous experience, the assumptive narrative goes, Cuencanos would surely start caring about what they are eating and the consequences of such consumption and change their behaviours. This resonates with Guthman's (2011) critical discussion of the causes and consequences of obesity, in which she stresses the problematic ways that neoliberal governmentality shifts responsibility away from public institutions onto the individual. Consumerist and educational approaches towards foods are thus favoured, and 'problems' located in a lack of personal responsibility and knowledge. Guthman thereby elucidates the politics of knowledge production and the manner it not only creates a problem to care about (and proffers a solution), but does so in a way that enables a particular group to 'socially scold' (ibid.: 18) an Other, concluding that 'the alternative-food movement attaches political citizenship and ethics to personal investments in body and health' (ibid.: 193).

In Cuenca we can see these dynamics of political citizenship and personal responsibility unfolding through the notion of privileged migrants caring about the diets and the bodies of Cuencanos. As their comments indicate, Cuencano eating preferences present a 'pedagogical moment' (Goodman, in press) through which the local population can learn to make 'better' food choices. Cuencanos thus need to learn, as far as privileged migrants are concerned, to care (more) about their food. And, to do so, they need to acquire knowledge about their preferred foods' 'dangers' in order to travel 'as far along as us'. As such, this discourse draws attention to Cuencanos' (assumed) lack of care, not only for themselves but also for society. They appear, following Guthman, to be lacking in political citizenship. It is important to note, however, that this absence is not necessarily seen as wilful and a form of neglect, but is instead premised on a (perceived) lack of knowledge and understanding. In turn, caring about what the locals eat can be understood as a demonstration of privileged migrants' own knowledge and global citizenship. It is not only their knowledge that matters here, however, but also their experience, action and personal responsibility. Privileged migrants, the narrative goes, have lived and eaten in a (Western) context of complex and 'dangerous' foods and have witnessed the 'dangers' first-hand, only to realize these and change their lives accordingly. They have learnt about what constitutes careful eating. To put it crudely, they have been there and have emerged on the other side whereas the local population, according to them, have not and are, moreover, not in a position to do so – or at least not to do so *yet*. As Xenia testifies, Cuencanos are still embracing complex foods without due care as it is still new to them; they have yet to learn what comprises careful eating.

There is consequently a time and spatial politics to privileged migrants caring about Cuencano eating practices, as they look back to – and arguably down upon – the local population with the benefit of their own hindsight based on (previously) being in a time and place in which complex foods are deeply embedded. I have argued previously that these individuals regard their move to Cuenca as a shift in time as well as space as they attempt to, somewhat misguidedly, return to a location that is, in the words of one, 'like living in the 1950s' (Abbots 2013: 121). I wish to extend this here and suggest that privileged migrants position not just the place of Cuenca, but also the Cuencanos contained within it as being further back in time, despite the latter's preference for 'modern' foods. How and what Cuencanos eat becomes a marker of this temporal distance, with the local population consuming industrial and modern foods because, in the words of Donna, they are a 'novelty'. Modernity thus belies a naivety. In contrast, privileged migrants construct themselves as having recognized the dangers of such developments and are now looking to 'return' – from a position further along the 'stream of time' (Fabian 1983: 17) – to a pre-industrialized situation where foods are 'simple'.

Caring about what others eat, then, can be seen as a mechanism through which these social distinctions are realized. I address the issues of nostalgia and the rendering of (a particular group) of Cuencanos into a past further below, but first I wish to highlight that it is not solely through imaginations of the past and present that social distance is created. Visions of a future also play a role, with privileged migrants constructing Cuencano eating preferences as predicated on gratification in the present and lacking foresight. Again, this highlights a (perceived) absence of Cuencano care about the longer-term consequences of their eating preferences, whereas privileged migrants' own cares about food in the present are orientated towards, and premised on, the future. As their comments testify, privileged migrants care about the longer-term implications of consuming complex food on the health of both individual and social bodies, as well as the natural environment. These cares are multi-faceted and there is slippage between a range of pressing and prescient concerns, with issues such as the level of obesity and associated health risks, waste, pollutants, food safety and pathogen levels, environmental damage, climate change, the erosion of culture, the demise of tradition and global homogenization all being raised by my participants to a greater or lesser extent. Moreover, it is not uncommon for the lines between these factors, and between caring-for and caring-about (Ungerson 1983; Tronto 1993) to be blurred, with privileged migrants – as can be seen in Angela's comment – associating the eating of processed foods and refined carbohydrates with a variety of social ills. Caring-for Cuencanos and their bodily health is, in this context, tantamount to caring about society, and its resilience and reproduction, more generally.

We Care (and Others Don't)

My point here is that there is no one easy answer to the question of why privileged migrants care about what Cuencanos eat. Instead, care is mobilized in, and takes on, a number of different guises, while frequently being packaged and crystallized around one issue (and solution). Spatially, it also extends beyond the local population and environs and is orientated to broader, more global concerns, such as the expansion of the global fast-food chains and the eradication of local culture. Again, this is another point of contrast with Cuencanos, who are commonly understood by privileged migrants as not only focused on immediate gratification but also as failing to recognize the effects of their eating preferences on the wider, global population. Thus, privileged migrants 'other' Cuencanos through the rubric of care and lack thereof. This arguably enables the former to construct a position of cultural authority over the latter. Yet, while they discursively create distance, the political and cultural capital of privileged migrants is limited outside of their specific social group, and they have little to no opportunity to influence, or interfere (Rousseau 2012), with the eating practices of the local population. They may be alternatively – and simultaneously – concerned and dismissive of Cuencano eating practices, but they can only be so from the sidelines of society. Nevertheless, their discourse – and the distancing it produces – provides a central tenet of their own self-identity.

As caring-for local bodies and caring-about what they eat is symptomatic of migrants' wider and deeply entrenched concerns about modernity and the globalization and industrialization of food, it is perhaps not surprising that discourses of food politics circulate widely and frequently in privileged migrant circles. One of the characteristics of these discussions that initially most surprised me was not just the frequency of food as a conversational topic, but also the uniformity of opinion and values. I am not saying here that migrants are a homogenous group, for tensions do exist within the community and migrants come from myriad social and economic backgrounds and have a range of political ideals and level of interaction with each other. Rather, I am suggesting that a contrary view on eating, for example that fast food chains were not necessarily as dangerous or as antithetical to ideas of good food as commonly represented, is a significant marker of difference which aligns one, perhaps, more closely to Cuencanos. At times I presented this and other 'alternative' views, with the aim of playing devil's advocate, and was met with anything from forceful rebuttals and personal rebukes to being frozen out of conversations. This suggests that caring about food (through a very particular lens) can be a mechanism through which privileged migrants forge relationships with each other through their shared ideals; care emphasizes their own similarities and proximities and minimizes their differences and distances.

Privileged migrants therefore tend to regard their own food preferences as both more caring and careful than the local population. Yet this enactment of care is not just directed towards Other people and places. Self-care is also inherently bound-up with their eating preferences, as they look to care for their own bodily health through the consumption of simple food and the avoidance of complexity and its associated risks. This, however, gives rise to tensions as caring for the self and caring for and about Others are not easily reconcilable (see also Lavis, this volume). In Cuenca, acquiring 'trustworthy' simple food that is also deemed 'safe' for their bodies results in many migrants avoiding local food sites, such as markets, and paradoxically acquiring their food from larger scale, industrial providers such as supermarket chains, as well as importing their own specialist health food products from the USA (Abbots 2013). The ironies of this, and contradictions between ideals and practice, is not lost on a number of my research participants who struggled to come to terms with their own practices and ventured towards 'unsafe' food in a bid to live the simple life they had imagined. Yet the issue remains that they find it difficult to care as they wish and, upon being presented with the dilemma of choosing self-care and large scale complexities that they consider are dangerous to society or practising their cares for society and opting for small-scale simple food that carries a risk to their own body, they ultimately select the former. A number sought to explain this decision on the grounds that an Ecuadorian supermarket chain is a less dangerous entity than a global fast food chain. They may well be correct, and no doubt many would concur, and I am not intent on staking a claim for either. What I do want to highlight, however, is that in making this argument, privileged migrants continue to show that while they do not – and cannot – care as much as they would like, they care more than the care-less Cuencanos who continue to eat processed, modern and industrial foods.

The Governing Classes: Caring About Cultural Continuities

Privileged migrants are not the only actors to care about the eating practices of the local population, nor in coalescing multiple, broader cares around the 'undesirable' food preferences of a particular social group. The actions of the local governing classes invoke striking parallels with privileged migrant discourse – and the culpable actors upon which it centres. Yet this group has arguably more political capital and leverage than the recently arrived privileged migrants, and their cares, as I aim to show, take on a more interventionist and governmental tone. In Cuenca city and its immediate suburbs, caring-for citizens takes the form of healthy eating education stalls in central locations, such as those near schools, parks and plazas, which reproduce normative clinical knowledge (for example, consume more fresh fruit and vegetables). In rural areas, however, these 'caring events' tend to take a different form and healthy eating education morphs into celebrations of local 'traditional' foods – known colloquially as *comida típica*[2] – often with accompanying history lessons and the championing of cultural continuities.

A health fair in Jima, a large village approximately an hour and a half bus journey away from Cuenca city, was one such caring event. The people of Jima, like many of the rural communities in the greater Cuencano region, have been feeling the effects of sustained, primarily male, migration to the United States and parts of Europe[3] and, in particular, members of the lower rural classes have been enjoying a new remittance-fuelled prosperity that has transformed their social and economic lives. As a consequence, their diet and eating preferences have inclined towards the processed and those foods deemed 'modern'. My research participants, who were predominantly drawn from this social group (hereafter the migrant-peasantry), commonly consumed refined carbohydrates and sugars in the form of white bread, white rice, soft drinks and added sugar juices, and ate little fresh fruit and vegetables. Their rural location prohibits their patronage of the global fast-food chains, although they commonly enjoy basted chicken and hotdog sausages from local fast-food restaurants and stalls. In short, their diet appears, at first glance, to be not that far removed from the stereotype created by privileged migrants and could be deemed as lacking in care, for both self and others, from this normative vantage point. Moreover, as the import of small-scale agriculture diminishes as an economic strategy, smallholdings make way for large villas, and the wealthiest employ domestic servants, leisure time has increased substantially and rural households have shifted from being units of production to ones of consumption (Abbots 2012a; Pribilsky 2007).

Jima's Health Fair, then, had the seemingly dual, and not necessarily compatible, aims of providing professional health support and caring for the rural lower classes whilst concomitantly celebrating local food. To this end, a health outreach vehicle, with accompanying professionals, dominated much of the affair and offered advice and pragmatic support on issues of body weight, nutrition, and diabetes, amongst other medical concerns. Running alongside this was a number of temporary food stalls, managed by the governing classes and run by the migrant-peasantry, which sold a range of 'healthy' dishes. These had to follow particular guidelines that were sensitive to the fair's theme and, consequently, the sale of hamburgers, fries, soft drinks and lager was banned. As one of my migrant-peasant participants, Sonia, explained to me, 'it's because they're not good for you, for

2   I have discussed *comida típica* and its mutable definitions at length elsewhere (Abbots 2011, 2012b, 2014a) but the term can loosely be translated to 'typical food of the region'.

3   See Abbots (2012a, 2014a) for further discussion, especially in relation to gender roles, labour relations, kinship and consumption practices. Also Miles (2004) and Pribilsky (2007) for ethnographic discussions of neighbouring communities, and Whitten (2003) for an overview of the transformative causes and consequences of migration in the region.

your body, they have a lot of fat'. However, her follow-up comment suggests another factor informed the guidelines; 'and it's because they're foods that aren't from here – they're from the USA'. In contrast, the foods that she and others were selling – roast guinea pig, *mote*, *empanadas* (deep fried cheese pastries) and *chicha* (maize fermented beer) – were 'from here'. One does not have to be a nutritionist to note that these foods are also high in fat and refined carbohydrates, and could also be classified as 'unhealthy' if one so desired. But, it appeared the governing class organizers were not desirous to do so, and placed the two types of foods into two very different categories – one that was unacceptable to the health fair and seen to be exogenous to the region, and the other acceptable and local.

In constructing this differentiation, the governing classes indicate the wider cultural values and political dynamics that inform their notions of caring and careful food. Specifically, their categorization of foods points to the ways in which the promotion of cultural continuities and concerns over disruption to traditions are bound up with the enactment of care, in this case for the bodily health of the (lower-class) individual. In other words, the health fair appears, at first glance, to be a caring intervention designed to improve the physical wellbeing of the rural lower classes in the face of increasing body mass and rises in related health concerns. But scratch beneath the surface and we start to see the valorization and promotion of local food heritage. This is not to negate the primary objective of the fair, or the work of the health professionals involved. I am merely arguing that there are other dynamics running alongside these caring interventions, and in this context they are the reproduction of 'tradition' in the form of *comida típica*. This process became even more visible when the fair's other activities commenced. These included a cookery competition, which was based on *comida típica* dishes and involved a number of participants dressed up in the costume of the *Chola Cuencana*. A history lesson followed this, in which the head teacher of the secondary school exhorted the gathered villagers not to forget their past, their origins, or their cooking traditions.

Teaching the Care-less Peasantry to Care

Jima's Health Fair indicates the extent that the governing classes echo privileged migrants' perspectives on globalization and industrialization, with these being regarded as irrevocably damaging to cultural continuities. The shifting food preferences and increasing body mass of the lower classes are seen as evidential of this perceived 'danger' and measures are subsequently taken to reinstate and promote a more 'traditional' diet. *Comida típica*, and the people who consume it, are thereby constructed as somewhat vulnerable to the exogenous influences of global fast-food chains and the industrial food system, in part because they are seen to not know any better and are thereby constructed as not in a position to fully care – for both themselves and about the consequences of their food preferences. They are, to all intents and purposes, regarded as caring less about such matters than those above them on the social scale. In reality, the eating practices of the migrant-peasantry are more resilient than they are given credit and *comida típica* is a rather flexible and dynamic category that allows for historical processes of colonization and creolization (Abbots 2011, 2012b, 2014b). But what emerges from this governing class discourse is: first how eating certain foods (and abstaining from others) is constructed as a mechanism of caring for culture and its reproduction; secondly, the extent that this discourse is targeted towards a particular social group; and thirdly, how education and knowledge are seen as a solution for this perceived absence of care. For while the governing classes may be orchestrating events like the Jima Health Fair, it is not their eating practices – or indeed their bodies – which are the concern here, despite them also frequenting global fast food chains, cosmopolitan cafés and fusion restaurants in the city (Abbots 2014b). Instead, it is those of the migrant-peasantry.

So why are the migrant-peasantry singled out for such 'caring' interventions? And why is this group discursively constructed as particularly care-less of their own corporeal and social body? The answer lies, in part, I argue in the general context of the transformation of social life witnessed in villages like Jima, where the established class hierarchies are being challenged by new remittance prosperity. This has led to the production and circulation of a discourse that extends beyond food practices in which the *nouveau riche* migrant-peasantry are publicly chastized and ridiculed for their 'naïve' and 'foolish' economic strategies and consumption practices that are, the narrative goes, creating a variety of social ills and breakdown. But is also relates, I contend, to the manner in which the bodies of peasants are inherently bound up in notions of local food and its (re)production.

'The peasantry', whether migrant or otherwise, have a unique position in that they are materially and discursively embedded in the food landscape as producers, as well as consumers. Moreover, the form of small-scale production with which they are associated is the very type of seemingly non-industrialized, non-complex and synchronic practices that are valued by privileged migrants and the governing classes alike. I am not saying here that these forms of production are timeless and simple, and my participants who maintained smallholdings used a variety of established techniques, such as oxen-pulled ploughs and planting during a full moon, alongside chemical fertilisers and modified seed. Rather I am arguing that privileged migrants and the governing classes attempt to gloss over historical processes and contemporary changes by constructing the peasantry, and their food practices, as bastions of 'tradition'.[4] A similar process has been located in Alentajo, Portugal by West and Domingos (2012), in reference to the Serpa cheese Presidia of the Slow Food Movement. They argue that, rather than challenging consumerism *per se*, such initiatives construct, through an elitist and middle-

---

4   Elsewhere I have discussed how these processes play out and are concomitantly contested and upheld by members of the migrant-peasantry, as well as unpacking the gendered dimensions of these dynamics (Abbots 2014a).

class valuing of 'tradition', notions of good and bad foods. As such, a narrative of the artisan local producer is created that glosses over historical political and economic relations and social change. Likewise, Brass' (2000) account of new social movements traces the intellectual genealogy of the agrarian myth and shows that primacy is given to tradition, culture and practices that are already seen to exist. Thus, peasantness is essentialized in a reactionary and regressive manner that can suppress grassroot voices in its attempt to recapture and rediscover an imaginary 'golden age'. Being a producer of 'simple' food does not, of course, equate to being such a consumer, and the peasantry have, by definition, historically produced for the market (Bernstein 2010). Yet, there is, I suggest, a collapsing of production and consumption within this privileged migrant/governing class discourse, in which assumptions are made about the eating preferences of the contemporary migrant-peasantry, based on nostalgic romanticized imaginations of 'the peasantry'. In short, because they are seen to have historically produced food in a 'traditional' manner, there is also an expectation that they eat in a 'traditional' way – and will continue to do so. More importantly in the context of this volume, they are expected to care about their food and its continuities. When they are perceived to not be doing so – to be careless – their eating practices are constructed as a problem that requires intervention and governance (cf. Foucault 1978).

These interventions take various forms ranging from explicit public critique in the local media to more subtle governance measures, including calls for tighter regulation to curtail the transformation of agricultural land and limit the construction of villas and expansion of non-productive spaces, such as leisure gardens. Moreover, those members of the migrant-peasantry, like Sonia, who refuse to perform their expected 'producer and purveyor of traditional food' role appear to be excluded from a number of community initiatives, especially those that promote a particular rural and cultural aesthetic to the tourist industry (Abbots 2014a). In addition, small-scale farming is high on the curriculum of rural schools. The school in Jima, for example, had a large plot and I witnessed schoolchildren working it and growing typical foods, such as corn, nearly every day. Luisa, a secondary school teacher who had worked in the city and its rural environs, talked me through recent national and local government initiatives that were promoting small-scale agriculture and explained how education was a key aspect of this programme. She told me:

> There is a national curriculum, but there is flexibility. The schools in the *campo*, they specialize much more in agriculture. It's because we don't have the skills anymore, since migration, and the *campesinos* don't know how to grow things. But the parents, they don't want their children to be associated with the *campo*, to learn those types of things.

Taken together, then, this raft of governing class led activities and initiatives, from health fairs and public history lessons to building regulations and agricultural education are orientated towards maintaining continuities in the food practices of the migrant-peasantry, upholding cultural traditions and reasserting established social roles. All invoke care in different guises, whether it is for bodily health in the case of the Health Fair, the landscape and rural aesthetic in reference to building regulations, or national agricultural yields and children's futures. Yet, despite these different ambitions, they all have a similar consequence of governing migrant-peasant bodies by looking to influence what and how they acquire food and what and how they eat. Moreover, they all discursively work to construct the migrant-peasantry as lacking in care. In turn, this (constructed) absence is defined as a problem that requires rectification and intervention; a process that consequently, following Foucault (1978), legitimizes the actions and authority of the governing classes.

A Care-Less Migrant-Peasantry?

> These things aren't important; we don't even think about them; it doesn't matter to us; people don't care where it [their food] comes from.

The above quotation comes from Juliana, a young lower class, but aspiring, Cuencana who grew up in the *campo* but now lives and works in Cuenca city. We were discussing the fast food industry specifically, and food safety and security more widely, following newspaper coverage of a recent 'discovery' of an illegal slaughterhouse in a small town outside Cuenca that had introduced horsemeat into the food chain. She continued to tell me that 'everyone in the area' knew about the slaughterhouse and it had only hit the headlines following ministerial involvement and an investigation by high-ranking government officials. She was also fairly ambivalent and pragmatic about such matters and unconcerned that horsemeat had been passed off as another type of meat, explaining that 'this happens all the time; you ask for a certain amount of beef, and they don't have it, so they give you the amount that is there and then make up the rest with meat from under the counter'. Moreover, she did not care that various types of meat were going onto the pile – 'cats, dogs, rats: anything they would find they would use'. For Juliana, her main issue was that the animals were unhealthy and that their diseases could cross-contaminate and enter the food chain as it had, according to her, ended up everywhere, 'especially in *embutidos* (processed meat products) – even those from [a European style chain popular with privileged migrants and the middle classes]'.

Juliana's views on meat appear to be a striking contrast, with the exception of the issue of food safety and personal bodily health, to those held by privileged migrants[5] and, as such, they lend credence to the widely held perception that the lower classes do not care about their food. In many respects, this discourse, although rarely based on intimate acquaintance as far as privileged migrants are concerned, seems to be a rather accurate summation. Juliana regaled to me on

---

5   And also those of Coles' participants (this volume).

another occasion how she was 'different' to many people of her social group because she knew about food and where it came from, due to her experience of working in one of the global chains:

> I know that the food for Cuenca is shipped from a centre, and the chickens are all kept in little tight cages, with the lights on all the time, and all they do is eat and eat so they get fat and have short little legs because they can't move and they're too heavy. But *other* people here don't; they just think the chicken comes from the *campo* like any other chicken and is killed there and then. (my emphasis)

The knowledge Juliana has does not stop her eating at the global chains, not least because of the opportunities to gain prestige and social status these restaurants offer an aspiring Cuencana and, in this way, her approach differs to that of privileged migrants. Nonetheless there are also parallels in the way she positions herself as knowledgeable of such food supply networks whereas Other people are not.

Juliana's views were widely supported by a number of my migrant-peasant participants, who also consistently made it known to me that they were not interested in where their food originated or how it was produced. The terms 'organic', 'fair trade' and 'higher welfare', for example, were not in their lexicon: an indication, perhaps, of the cultural specificity of such labels (see Coles this volume). It is tempting to attribute this seeming lack of care to a range of other absences including the lack of visibility and prevalence of such labels, a lack of alternative food movements and associated discourses, a lack of choices available to consumers, and a lack of resources through which to obtain such foods. Notwithstanding, I would better reflect, perhaps, the perspectives of my participants if I did not try to explain away their lack of interest (or care) through structural factors and simply reiterated Juliana's statement that 'these things aren't important' to them.

To define lower class rural Cuencanos approach to food as essentially non-caring and care-less would, however, be a misrepresentation. Caring is not just a practice to which they are subjected, and potentially challenge through their continued consumption of complex and industrially processed foods in the face of the governance and education measures and the public critique of privileged migrants and the governing classes. They also enact care relations through food and, despite all appearances to the contrary, can also care about foods' origins, albeit on a different scale and in a more private and intimate context. In so doing, they too create relations of distance and proximity and establish sameness and otherness.

Kinship Relations: Creating Otherness through Intimacies

Cuy (guinea pig) is a dish that is lavished with a great deal of care, as well as being a mechanism through which care is enacted. It is also a dish commonly defined as *comida típica* and consequently celebrated as cultural heritage by the governing classes in events such as the Jima Health Fair. But members of the migrant-peasantry do not need to be taught to care about *cuy*, or for its cultural continuities for that matter, as it remains deeply embedded in their domestic and intimate lives, and their self-care of their households. *Cuy* has been noted to have a unique capacity to create and maintain social bonds (Abbots 2011; Bourque 2001; Weismantel 1988). It is an exceptional foodstuff in that its consumption, with some omissions like the Jima Health Fair[6], is restricted to public and private festive occasions and shared only within close social networks. Moreover, its production and preparation are characterized by a labour-intensive, non-mechanized and time-consuming process. In short, it is a dish firmly associated with commensality, sociality, intimacy and the making of individuals as kin (cf. Carsten 1997). In Jima's migratory context this takes on an additional dimension, as packages of the roast dish are sent from women in Jima to their male kin living in New York, effectively remaking them 'Jimeño' and minimizing loss (Abbots 2011). What is of import here, for both sender and receiver alike, is that the *cuy* 'tastes of home', with migrants asserting that those acquired from elsewhere do not have the same unique flavour as those received from their kin. This is because, according to my participants, other, more commercially available, *cuyes* did not receive the same level of attention and care as those raised and prepared by kin, nor are they composed with the same materials as those 'from home'. As Rosa explained:

> It's to do with what the *cuyes* eat. I don't know what other *cuyes* from *other* places eat, or what people feed them, but it's a mixture of things. But good *cuy*, should eat alfalfa and *hierba* (local grass), that's what makes them good for eating.

In this context, unlike chicken and other meat discussed by Juliana above, origins are important and the migrant-peasantry care where *cuy* comes from. This is because, I suggest, for the particular dish of *cuy* to make a person Jimeño (or Cuencano) it has to be from Jima (or Cuenca). The natural resources of the place – in the form of feed – are materially transformed into the meat of the *cuy*, which, in turn, is digested and constitutes the body of the eater. Lavishing care on the *cuy* can thus be translated into caring for the person who will be eating it, especially when the person in question is physically absent as is the case in this migratory context. This, in turn, promotes kin and cultural continuities.

This form of feeding and eating appears to be somewhat benign, and related more to social closeness and the creation of intimacies, which is how I have previously framed the consumption and exchange of *cuy* (Abbots 2011). This resonates with the established literature on commensality and the biological and emotional incorporation of individuals into a social group through the ingestion of

---

6   On such occasions, measures are taken to personally distance the producer/preparer from the meat and minimize intimacies (Abbots 2014a).

shared substances (Carsten 1997). But I now want to consider the flipside of the process. Holtzman (2013) reminds us of this and the ways in which closeness can be stifling and family relations fraught (see also Wilk 2010). Hence, the tensions within these intimate surroundings should also be considered, and that which seems apolitical and benign may, indeed, be wracked with political dynamics. The act of giving, and withholding, food has a power dimension in that it subjects a body to the actions of an Other, a contention examined by Weismantel (1988) in an Ecuadorian context who demonstrates that the serving of food provides women with a sense of empowerment in an otherwise patriarchal society. As such, accepting food can be regarded as an act of voluntary subjugation to an Other and an acknowledgement of their (not uncommonly temporary and transient) authority. Returning to Jima and the migrant-peasantry, we see a similar relation in the practice of sending packages of *cuy* to migrated kin. On one hand, this can be regarded as an act of caring for physically absent loved ones and a token of ongoing affection. But on the other, it can be seen as a practice of governance, through which Jimeña women enact and maintain their authority within their distributed household, and ensure that their continued presence is felt through the foods they send and encourage their migrated male kin to ingest. Caring through feeding can consequently be regarded as an act of governance through which individuals inscribe themselves onto the body of Others. As such, they establish a dynamic of distance and differentiation while simultaneously creating closeness. Caring-for others, therefore, can be – and is – a nurturing and loving act that facilitates proximity. But is also one that enables the construction of otherness, even in the most intimate of domains.

Conclusion

In this chapter I have traversed myriad ways through which otherness is produced through the entangled dynamics of eating and caring. These processes are situated at multiple scales and located within a range of social relations: within migrant peasant households, between the governing classes and the migrant-peasantry and between privileged migrants and the local Cuencano population. In so doing, I have drawn attention the ways in which individuals and social groups look to demonstrate that they care not only through their eating practices, but also their judgement of others'. As such, I have sought to show how care can be deployed and mobilized as a political tool that helps establish and maintain social distance, even in the most intimate of settings.

Care is a slippery concept that takes many different forms and guises. Moreover, it is also a concept that wraps and shrouds political dynamics: it is premised on taken-for-granted notions of what is good for self and society such as, in this context, cultural continuities, bodily health and local foods. However, it is this very shrouding, and the ease with which care is manipulated, that gives care its political and problematic characteristic. In the greater Cuencano region to ostensibly care-for Others is to care-about a range of wider concerns. However, in caring, I have contended, privileged migrants and the governing classes discursively construct Others – the local Cuencano population and the migrant-peasantry – as lacking in care. This (assumed) absence, in turn, is produced as a problem that requires interventionist measures that concomitantly, following Foucault (1978), legitimize the social authority of particular cares and carers and help minimize social distance between them while simultaneously establishing distance between self and the Other. In the light of such interventions, it is tempting to regard the migrant-peasantry's and Cuencano individuals' continued consumption of 'bad' foods – or their lack of care – as an embodied challenge to such governance attempts. There is danger, however, of overlaying conscious political action onto practices about which individuals claim they 'do not care'. Hence I am somewhat cautious in attempting to make such an argument, although I would like to raise the possibility that to not care, or to not demonstrate care in ways that are socially expected, is a form of appropriation and contestation of dominant discourses of what constitutes careful eating.

Whether or not Cuencanos and the migrant-peasantry care about what and how they eat is subject to question and in this chapter I have tried to tease out other ways that the enactment of care *vis-à-vis* eating can be glimpsed while also being faithful to my participants' own voices that they do not care about such matters. However, we should, perhaps, not be asking how much people care about what they eat, but where their caring relations are directed and how they are enacted through their eating practices. Moreover, we need to ask what 'to care' means and what forms it can take in particular social contexts for particular individuals and social groups, as well as what care does. Only then, I suggest, can we start to understand the ways that care – as both practice and sentiment – can be politically deployed as a governance tool.

Acknowledgements

The research on which this chapter is based was part funded by a Wenner Gren Foundation post PhD grant. My appreciation goes to all my research participants who so generously shared their time and knowledge with me during my periods of fieldwork in Ecuador. My thanks also to Mike Goodman and Ben Coles, as well as my co-editors, for their helpful comments on earlier drafts. All errors and omissions remain, however, my own.

References

Abbots, E-J. 2011. 'It doesn't taste as good from the pet shop': Guinea pig consumption and the performance of class and kinship in Highland Ecuador and New York City. *Food, Culture and Society*, 14(2), 205-24.

Abbots, E-J. 2012a. In the absence of men? Gender, migration and domestic labour in the southern Ecuadorean Andes. *Journal of Latin American Studies*, 44(1), 71-96.

Abbots, E-J. 2012b. The celebratory and the everyday: Guinea pigs, hamburgers and the performance of food heritage in Highland Ecuador, in *Celebrations: The Proceedings of the Oxford Symposium on Food and Cookery 2011*, edited by M. McWilliams. London: Prospect Books, 12-23.

Abbots, E-J. 2013. Negotiating foreign bodies: Migration, trust and the risky business of eating in Highland Ecuador, in *Why We Eat, How We Eat: Contemporary Encounters Between Foods and Bodies*, edited by E-J. Abbots and A. Lavis. Farnham: Ashgate, 119-38.

Abbots, E-J. 2014a. The fast and the fusion: Class, creolization and the remaking of *comida típica* in Highland Ecuador, in *Food Consumption in Global Perspective. Essays in the Anthropology of Food in Honour of Jack Goody*, edited by J. Klein and A. Murcott. Basingstoke: Palgrave Macmillan, 87-107.

Abbots, E-J. 2014b. Embodying country-city relations: The figure of the *Chola Cuencana* in Highland Ecuador, in *Food Between the Country and the City: Ethnographies of a Changing Global Foodscape*, edited by N. Domingos, J. Sobral and H.G. West. London: Bloomsbury, 41-57.

Barnes, M. 2012. *Care in Everyday Life: An Ethic of Care in Practice*. Bristol: Policy Press.

Bernstein, H. 2010. *Class Dynamics of Agrarian Change*. Sterling: Kumarian Press.

Bourque, N. 2001. Eating your words: Communicating with food in the Ecuadorian Andes, in *An Anthropology of Indirect Communication*, edited by J. Hendry and C.W. Watson. London: Routledge, 85-100.

Brass, T. 2000. *Peasants, Popularism and Postmodernism: The Return of the Agrarian Myth*. London: Frank Cass.

Carsten, J. 1997. *The Heat of the Hearth: The Process of Kinship in a Malay Fishing Community*. Oxford: Clarendon Press.

Fabian, J. 1983. *Time and the Other: How Anthropology Makes its Object*. New York: Columbia University Press.

Fechter, A-M. 2007. *Transnational Lives: Expatriates in Indonesia*. Aldershot, UK and Burlington, USA: Ashgate Publishing Ltd.

Foucault, M. 1978. *The History of Sexuality: An Introduction*. New York: Pantheon.

Goodman, M.K. In press. Afterword, in *Food Pedagogies*, edited by R. Flowers and E. Swan. Farnham: Ashgate.

Guthman, J. 2011. *Weighing In: Obesity, Food Justice, and the Limits of Capitalism*. Berkeley and Los Angeles, CA: University of California Press.

Holtzman, J. 2013. Reflections on fraught food, in *Why We Eat, How We Eat: Contemporary Encounters Between Foods and Bodies*, edited by E-J. Abbots and A. Lavis. Farnham: Ashgate, 139-146.

International Living Why Ecuador [online]. Available at: http://www.internationalliving.com/Countries/Ecuador/Why-Ecuador [accessed: 18 March 2010].

Miele, M. and Evans, A.B. 2010. When foods become animals: Ruminations on ethics and responsibility in care-full practices of consumption. *Ethics Place and Environment*, 13(2), 171-90.

Miles, A. 2004. *From Cuenca to Queens: An Anthropological Story of Transnational Migration.* Austin, TX: University of Texas Press.

Mol, A., Moser, I. and Pols, J. 2010. *Care in Practice: On Tinkering in Clinics, Homes and Farms.* New London: Transaction Publishers.

Ong, A. 1999. *Flexible Citizenship: The Cultural Logics of Transnationality.* Durham, NC: Duke University Press.

Pribilsky, J. 2007. *La Chulla Vida: Gender, Migration and the Family in Andean Ecuador & New York City.* Syracuse, NY: Syracuse University Press.

Rousseau, S. 2012. *Food Media: Celebrity Chefs and the Politics of Everyday Interference.* London: Berg.

Tronto, J. 1993. *Moral Boundaries: A Political Argument for an Ethic of Care.* London: Routledge.

Ungerson, C. 1983. Why do women care?, in *A Labour of Love: Women, Work and Caring*, edited by J. Finch and D. Groves. London: Routledge and Kegan Paul Books, 41-9.

Weismantel, M. 1988. *Food, Gender and Poverty in the Ecuadorian Andes* Philadelphia, PA: University of Pennsylvania Press.

Weismantel, M.J. 2001. *Cholas and Pishtacos: Stories of Race and Sex in the Andes.* Chicago, IL: University of Chicago Press.

Weismantel, M.J. 2003. Mothers of the *Patria*: La Chola Cuencana and La Mama Negra, in *Millennial Ecuador: Critical Essays on Cultural Transformations and Social Dynamics*, edited by N.E. Whitten. Iowa City: University of Iowa Press, 325-54.

West, H.G and Domingos, N. 2012. Gourmandizing poverty food: The Serpa cheese slow food presidium. *Journal of Agrarian Change*, 12(1), 120-43.

Whitten, N.E. 2003. Introduction, in *Millennial Ecuador: Critical Essays on Cultural Transformations and Social Dynamics*, edited by N.E. Whitten, Iowa City: University of Iowa Press, 1-45.

Wilk, R. 2010. Power at the table: Food fights and happy meals. *Cultural Studies: Critical Methodologies*, 10(6), 428-36.

PART II
Embodied Encounters
between Eating and Caring

Turning to focus on embodiment and corporeality, this central part interrogates encounters between food and care at the level of individual as well as social bodies. Acting as the analytic pivot between Parts I and III of the volume, it engages with the complex multi-directionality of relations between eating and caring, exploring how they diverge, overlap and take place at many scales. Tracing how knowledge claims and registers of value around eating frame, shape and enter into bodies, the contributors also explore eating as an act that resists or repositions such discourses, offering up alternative modalities of care and self-care. Across diverging empirical contexts they thereby challenge often taken-for-granted linkages between care, food and bodies, and take the body as the starting point from which to trace alternative relations engendered by both eating and caring.

The part begins by engaging with discourses of care that both shape but also emerge from the 'foodwork' of (not) eating practices in anorexia. These elucidate that seemingly disconnected flows of caring may simultaneously overlap as well as clash in the processual shaping of Selfhood and Otherness. It is also these convergences and entanglements that emerge when turning to interrogate the disconnect between discursive framings of refined sugar and the relational intimacies of ingesting sweet foods. Here we see that caring about what others eat in public health and biomedical discourses can eclipse the affective materialities of food and eating, as focus shifts towards the patrolling of body contours. By entering into clinical encounters that focus on weight, the part ends by drawing out this troubling of materiality, as both foods and bodies become quantifiable. Across these chapters, then, food emerges as a problematic vector that can be set to care in particular ways whilst obscuring or truncating others. All three contexts highlight interplays of absence and presence as eating and caring are seen to obscure as well as engender one another.

This part demonstrates, thus, that interactions between food and care are multiply sited, taking place within and between, as well as beyond, bodies. Their moments of encounter are lived and felt, and may be subjectively experienced as lacking in care. As such both eating and caring emerge as ways in which materialities, bodies and selves are produced and disrupted as well as mediated.

Chapter 4

Careful Starving: Reflections on (Not) Eating, Caring and Anorexia

Anna Lavis

Engaging with the volume's interrogation of what is 'brought to the table' by exploring interplays between care and food across diverse contexts, this chapter engages with the question: why and how does *not* eating engender or mobilize care? To explore this, it draws on data from two qualitative studies within large NHS inner-city mental health trusts in England: The first involved participant observation and interviews with service users in an eating disorders inpatient unit (2007-2008) and the second comprised interviews with users of eating disorders outpatient, daypatient and inpatient services (2013-2015). By engaging with individuals diagnosed with anorexia, alongside clinical and ethical discussions of treatment, this chapter traces how competing paradigms of caring and eating, illness and selfhood, touch edges in the bodies and lives of individuals living with anorexia. In so doing, it widens the question posed above to ask what food and care both *are* and *do* in the myriad moments of their embodied encounters.

In clinical terms, the self-starvation of anorexia nervosa is regarded as lacking in self-care and propelled by a loss of agency to the illness. This conceptualizes food not only as *the* vector through which to care for an individual with anorexia, but also as that which (re-)produces their self-care, where that comes to mean literally care of the self. Feeding (as eating through caring) is positioned as forging a teleological pathway from a current illness to a future anorexia-free self. In the clinic (see Foucault 2003) food is therefore 'an essential therapeutic intervention' (Powers and Cloak 2013: 82) not only for the integrity of the suffering body but also for the recovery of selfhood. However, engaging with individuals with anorexia elucidates not only how such care may be experienced as care-less, but also that embodied practices of not eating engender alternative modes of attention; anorexia, although recognized by participants as an illness, offers ways of caring both for oneself and for Others. Such caring through not eating maintains both anorexia and selfhood as the illness maps and matters the space of the present moment in ways that may render this endurable.

Reflecting on entanglements between food and care in anorexia, then, constitutes an argument for an analysis of anorexia that both engages with the lived vulnerabilities of material bodies whilst also going beyond a focus on emaciation as a goal of self-starvation (see also Gooldin 2008; Lavis 2013, 2014; Warin 2010). Yet, this is also not to ignore the enormous suffering that anorexia can cause or to regard practices of not eating as either fully agential or lacking in agency. There is no doubt that eating disorders are often, as Bob Palmer puts it, 'miserable and life blighting' (2014: iii) illnesses, but they also emerge from research participants' narratives as integral to selfhood. As such, the distress that anorexia causes is intertwined with individuals' ways of caring for self and Others both through and in spite of the illness. Exploring entanglements between food and care traces the texture and sociality of not eating practices, allowing anorexia's clinical realities to remain acknowledged but 'bracketed' (see Biehl and Locke 2010: 318) in order that other narratives may also be heard.

Central to this inquiry is the concept of 'foodwork'. This has previously been used in relation to the feeding practices that are part of caregiving in clinical/ residential settings, such as with individuals with dementia (cf. Heaven et al. 2013; Pierson 1999). In that context, foodwork's meaning is shaped by the analogous term, 'bodywork'; this has been described as the 'ambivalent, hidden work that tends to remain unarticulated within official discourses' of care (Twigg 2006: 136. See also Mol et al. 2010b). Recognizing bodywork as the conceptual underpinning of foodwork highlights the emotional labour and boundary-crossing intimacies of caring for another's body in feeding as much as in other activities such as washing (cf. Twigg 2002; Pols 2013). As such, whilst holding firmly within its parameters a sense of how eating and feeding may be vectors of care, the concept of foodwork also highlights the potential tensions and regimes of value embedded in such mobilizations of caring. Foodwork is thereby a productive concept; it allows us to hold together in one analytical space the (not) eating practices of individuals with anorexia, which we might term careful eating, and the feeding practices of the clinic, which we could term care-full feeding. Exploring each of these as diverse modalities of foodwork offers insights into ways in which performances of caring *about* and *for* (Fisher and Tonto 1990) entangle food and bodies, and comprise both emotional labour and value constructions.

Yet, while these modalities of caring may sometimes clash, sometimes co-exist and often 'map onto different dimensions' (Mol 2010: 217), there are also convergences between the clinic and individuals with anorexia. Although the chapter begins with mobilizations of eating through caring on the eating disorders unit (EDU), and goes on to explore how individuals' practices of not eating mobilize alternative pathways of caring, the flows of directionality are not so neat; these entanglements between food and care do not overlay the two empirical contexts in such a binary way. It is particularly in paying attention to shifting positionings of the body that overlaps and mimeses emerge. Food, bodies and care are all negotiated in relation to one another. Foodwork therefore emerges as a 'complex and embodied activity' (Pierson 1999: 130) on the part of the clinic and research participants whilst also being related to bodily materialities and embodiment in uncertain ways. Diverging conceptualizations of anorexia(s) and selves enacted through food and care produce, as well as intervene in, particular bodies. As such, this chapter echoes Annemarie Mol by asking, 'what kind of matter is food? What kinds of bodies does it feed?'(Mol 2012: 2), and suggests that care offers a productive way to explore these questions.

The Clinic: Anorexia *and* Care

Self-starvation is arguably central to a diagnosis of anorexia nervosa, and the illness is regarded as underpinned by 'an intense fear of gaining weight or becoming fat' (American Psychiatric Association 2013). That an individual with anorexia often 'neither gives up in the face of the negative consequences of eating restraint (not least hunger)' (Palmer 2014: 5) means that anorexia has 'one of the highest mortality rates of all psychiatric illnesses' (Bogle 2000: 2). Although 'most patients with anorexia nervosa receive treatment solely on an outpatient basis ... a substantial minority receive inpatient treatment' (NICE 2004: 6.5.2). It is suggested that 'patients may require inpatient care if they are suicidal or have life-threatening medical complications ... or weight below 85 percent of their healthy body weight' (Williams et al. 2008: 187).

Treatment can be enforced in England through sectioning under the mental health act 'where substantial risk cannot be managed in any other way' (NICE 2004: 6.5.7.3), although only 'a relatively low proportion of inpatients with anorexia nervosa are placed on formal compulsory treatment orders, with reports ranging from 9% to 28%' (Tan et al. 2010: 14). The justification for enforcing treatment is underpinned by framing individuals with anorexia as lacking the capacity to make decisions regarding treatment as a result of their compromised physical state (see Giordano 2005). On the other hand, scholars have argued that accepting an individual's treatment refusal can be ethical, especially if this is an autonomous decision against a background of frequent or repeated treatment failure (see Draper 2000; Matusek and Wright 2010). Attention on the part of medical ethicists in recent years to values, seeing these rather than individual autonomy as affected by the illness, has also challenged an assumed loss of capacity in anorexia, thereby furthering complexity (see Tan and Hope 2008). As such, anorexia and its care present to professionals a nexus of complex issues.

However, it has been suggested that if we accept that 'anorexia nervosa is not inevitably a progressive terminal illness ... it is preferable that treating physicians focus on the preservation of life' (Melamed et al. 2003: 62). Given the risks of severe emaciation and the 'intensive care' (Treasure and Schmidt 2005: 95) required by the starved body, it is clear how from a clinical point of view, 'there is no doubt that the appropriate treatment is food' (ibid.: 95). Thus, although guidelines state that 'weight gain is only one outcome of interest' (NICE 2004: paragraph 6.4.9), arguably 'the common goal is to re-feed the patient' (Griffiths and Russell 1998: 128), particularly in inpatient treatment. As such, although the heterogeneous nature of clinical practices must be acknowledged (see Berg and Mol 1998) with differing approaches existing alongside widespread recognition that psychological input is key, it is clear that food is a central vector of care.

Glimpsed through the regular weigh-ins of outpatient treatment, where food consumed since the last appointment is measured through the body, this caring through food is most starkly brought to the fore in daycare and inpatient treatment.

On the eating disorders inpatient unit (EDU) on which I conducted ethnographic fieldwork, meals are only one part of an extensive programme of psychological support. Yet a pervasive focus on feeding structures the temporal rhythms of the unit as all other activities, from recreation to therapy, are arranged around mealtimes. If I bumped into someone I had not seen for a few hours and asked them what they 'had been up to,' many would reply with humour, 'eating!' As one participant, Kate[1], put it, 'every day is just, sort of, eating, to be honest … . My whole life is planned around meals'. Likewise, in her interview, Abigail said:

> They [staff] always tell us 'you have to eat, it's normal'. Oh yeah, cos, everyone has a sandwich an hour after they've had lunch! … All they do in inpatient treatment is feed you, food, food, food, more food … I wish they'd admit that all they do is feed you and then let you go. I just wish they'd admit that, or warn you that's what's going to happen when you go in. They say they're going to change you and … and help and stuff. But they don't, they just make you fatter. (Abigail, inpatient, 2008)

It frequently infuriated participants when staff would not admit that three meals and three Snacks amounting to 3,500 calories a day was, as one participant Chloe put it, 'a shed load of food'. Peter, a temporary psychiatric nurse charged with the task of watching over lunch on his first day on the unit exclaimed in a loud whisper to the service user eating next to him, 'gosh you really do have to eat a lot, don't you!' He was thoroughly chastised for this in a subsequent staff meeting but participants discussed how they 'appreciated his honesty,' which was contrasted to the discursive norms of the unit. These norms are twofold: On the one hand, as Abigail suggests, there is a framing of eating as 'normal'. On the other, when the amount of food was challenged by service users, staff would frequently move away from attempts at normalization to instead tell service users that 'whilst you're on the EDU, food is medicine' (see also Long et al. 2012). This discursive framing positions mealtimes as clinical events that transact a substance – medicine – to be taken for one's own good. In turn, any refusal to eat on the part of service users comes to be seen (and perhaps also felt by staff) as a refusal of their care.

On the EDU such refusals to eat, alongside vocalizations of distress at eating or desire to talk about food or weight on the part of service users were often described by staff as 'the anorexia talking' (see Tan 2003). This conceptualizes such articulations as ensuing from a loss of agency to anorexia and sees the illness as a current and temporary addendum to a patient's 'authentic self' (Bruch 1974; Tan 2003). It suggests that 'the individual doesn't really want to restrict her eating, lose weight, or resist treatment – her Real Self has been invaded/infected/

---

1   All names are pseudonyms.

colonized by an Outside Force' (Vitousek 2005: 3). Expounding such a clear division aims to encourage service users to externalize their anorexia and thereby re-find – literally recover – an illness-free self that is conceptualized not only as having become trapped in, or effaced by, anorexia, but also as having preceded it. What is advocated therefore is a change back into what one once was and, perhaps, *should* be again. This elucidates, as does this volume more widely, that 'caring is an activity in which (often moral) valuing is implied' (Heuts and Mol 2013: 130. See also Barnes 2012).

To claim that not eating, or refusing the caring-as-feeding on the EDU, on the part of an anorexic individual is not an autonomous or 'authentic' decision in this way does save lives. It forms part of the architecture that justifies enforcement of treatment under the mental health act, noted above. Yet, this not only is underpinned by a particular value-laden paradigm of selfhood and pathology but also offers a way in which to perform this as care; it cleaves a conceptual space between anorexia and self into which caring through food can be fitted. This – in relation to Fisher and Tronto's (1990) four dimensions of care – forges a pathway from 'caring *about*', framed as attentiveness, to 'Caring *for*', framed as the work of caring (see also Tronto 1993; Ungerson 1983). Eating thereby becomes the vector through which selfhood is rematerialized through the measurably-expanding body – literally dripped back in through the swallowing of every mouthful. The so-called 'authentic self' is at once the receiver and also goal of care, and is thereby positioned tensely within two temporalities at once. Food, likewise, is both the focus of this work, and also made to work in a particular way.

Exploring these feeding practices as a form of foodwork highlights how nutritional value takes precedence over any other aspect of the sticky materiality of food. As food becomes medicine, bodily perimeters likewise become linear markers of illness or health, whilst intimate trajectories of food through corporeal spaces are rendered paradoxically 'immaterial'; food as a vector of care does not 'matter' in and of itself. In their exploration of care and food in a nursing home, Harbers et al. (2002) show how food is constructed differently within ethical and medical discussions of food refusal and feeding in the context of dementia. A 'medical attitude to food (appreciating it for its nutritional value)' (ibid.: 216-17) is contrasted to an ethical paradigm of food as a 'means to an end: survival, that may be desirable or not' (ibid.: 217). On the EDU, as the nutritional value of food also becomes enfolded into survival as an end goal, these discourses merge to coalesce into one teleological production of food *as* care. Yet, not only is the sensory materiality of food missing from this, but so too perhaps is the lived experience of being cared for.

To suggest this is not to deny the care that is conducted in the clinic; participants invariably recognized its value for other service users if not for themselves. However, many also described the EDU as 'terrifying' and 'awful', with mealtimes the focus of their fear and distress (see also Eli 2014; Gremillion 2003). Harbers et al. argue that a caring attitude is one 'which tries to accommodate and please a person' (2002: 217). Arguably the EDU's foodwork, and its underpinning in 'the anorexia talking', dislocate both caring and eating from 'pleasing' not only in terms of the materialities of food but also of the person. The person, it is suggested, is currently absent as the present is *filled* only with anorexia, which must be replaced by food. As such, the anorexia of the *present* is worked on through foodwork in order to teleologically care for the self of the *future*. If, then, care comprises sustained 'tinkering towards improvement' (Heuts and Mol 2013: 125. See also Mol et al. 2010a), it is clear that the EDU's foodwork does care but that it does so in a way that sees improvement as both in the future and in the body.

Foregrounding the feeding of the body as the central element of care serves to locate anorexia *in* the body. It is clear that the suffering body is arguably one of the few ways that anorexia can be clinically 'grasped' in order that individuals may be cared for and so this positioning is pragmatic. However, it also serves to make bodies *essentially anorexic* and anorexia *essentially bodily*. Bodies thus are arguably not only made in the literal sense of nourishment on the EDU, but also in a more conceptual way; the clinic maps a particular paradigm of anorexia through the corporeal depths of digestive geographies (see Willems 1998). It is against the background of this particular arrangement of self, body and anorexia performed by the clinic's ways of caring that we now turn to engage with narratives of individuals with anorexia. From these emerge alternative arrangements of anorexia and corporeality, illness and self.

Anorexia *as* Self-Care

In her interview Tammy recounted how her anorexia 'was never kind of a deliberate diet to lose weight or anything like that'. She said: 'it's never been so much of a body image problem for me, it was more just kind of not wanting to eat and kind of regaining control over that'. Tammy described how control was gained not only by ingesting as little as possible without dying, but also by an accompanying preoccupation with food that we might term 'virtual foodwork'. This was also apparent in Lacey's interview:

> I remember sitting on the bus on the way back from school ... And I got off the bus and I realized that I'd spent the entire bus journey counting the calories that I'd eaten that day, and that I was going to have to eat when I got home. And then I was thinking about the calories that I'd eaten all week and all that kinda stuff and it was like ... like looking back on that, it was just like I was thinking about probably so I don't have to think about everything else. (Lacey, daypatient, 2014)

I have explored elsewhere how practices, such as calorie counting and restricting food intake, which both enact and enframe *not* eating, illustrate that self-starvation does not simply constitute a lack in anorexia. Rather, it comprises continual work in order to engender 'relationships of absence' with food through which anorexia is processually maintained (Lavis 2013). The illness is therefore both dependent upon, but also of greater significance than, practices of not eating. As such, the foodwork of not eating here is, on the one hand, in opposition to that of the clinic. Yet these also share and set to work a conceptualization of food as quantifiable in a way that belies any sense of its sticky materiality. Above, I suggested this effacement in the clinic to be produced by the enfolding of a medical model of food into an ethical paradigm of saving lives. In participants' narratives now, food's materiality is again obscured in its intertwining with particular productions of value. However, these relate to the space of the present rather than future, as foodwork emerges as a way of producing anorexia to care for the self. This takes us beyond the clinic's binaries of self and Other, future and present.

In her interview, Josie, described her self-starvation and the virtual foodwork that accompanied it as:

> A distraction and an escape from the real world, the pressures, the worries, the stress, things that I couldn't control, things that I didn't know how to handle. It's a really easy thing to focus on and to let take up your mind … . It was something to focus on that didn't hurt, that I could control when I couldn't sort out some of the other issues. (Josie, inpatient, 2014)

That not eating offers a way of controlling and numbing emotions is recognized; anorexia has been described as 'a functional coping strategy in which control of eating serve[s] as a means of coping with ongoing stress and exerting control' (Eivors et al. 2003: 96. See also Treasure et al. 2007). Yet these accounts of 'counting calories', and thereby 'escap[ing] from the real world', also suggest that the numbness offered by virtual and actual self-starvation goes beyond the control of emotions. By letting anorexia 'take up your mind', as Josie put it, there would seem here to be an agential absenting of the self that both maps onto and yet importantly also contrasts with the conceptualizations of self and illness in the clinic, above. In her interview, Claudine said:

> You just sit there and sometimes it [anorexia] manifests itself in a sort of numbness and I'll just lie on my bed, stare into space and I'll sleep a lot or something like that. I just want to stop thinking and you do almost zone out as it were. (Claudine, inpatient, 2008)

In many participants' accounts there is a slippage between this zoning *out* through anorexia described by Claudine and the illness as a space to zone *into*. Anorexia was described by one participant as 'my space' and another as a 'my little bubble', with Emila saying 'it's almost like it's a world that you live in, that's separate from everybody else'. In her interview Nita described this spatiality in terms of safety. She said that anorexia had 'been a safety net for so long, removing it is the scariest thing in the world. … I think that's what has stopped me getting better completely and being fully recovered, is that it's a safety net that I don't want to remove'. She continued, 'it becomes so much a part of you' and asked, without it, 'what would I be?'

The sense here of anorexia as a 'safe space' that offers 'retreat' is reminiscent of Ellen Corin's discussions of 'positive withdrawal' (Corin 2007) in psychosis. Corin suggests that withdrawal signifies a way to 'defend an inner space' (ibid.: 283) through the construction of a kind of 'psychic skin that parallels the social skin' (ibid.: 283). Reflecting on anorexia as 'psychic skin' illustrates that the illness, as a space of numbness or retreat, is not empty; it does not comprise a gap where the 'authentic self' used to, or should, be. Rather, in participants' accounts anorexia stills the present in a way that forges an alternative subjectivity of space and being; this is a space *for* and *of* selfhood whilst also, importantly, being recognized as a space forged through illness. Yet, this is not to see the self simply as suspended or held within anorexia. Rather, selfhood 'manifests', to borrow Claudine's word, within and with the illness. Whilst poignantly elucidating how the cleaving attempts to remove anorexia from self on the part of the clinic may be experienced as care-less rather than care-full, Nita's questioning of 'what would I be' without anorexia, evinces an 'intersubjective fusion' (Jackson 2002: 340) with the illness that runs through many participants' narratives. Thus, if the foodwork of not eating processually maintains anorexia for participants, it also maintains their sense of self. In so doing, it is felt to be a modality of self-care that mediates how they live and move through the present moment.

Kate described anorexia as 'how I do things. You do it quietly, you do it on your own'. Likewise, Elisa said of anorexia that it 'would be probably the only thing in my life that's been constant for the last, I don't know, seven or eight years or something and I guess it's become a part of me and a part of my routine'. These descriptions of anorexia as 'part of my routine' and 'how I do things', afford a glimpse into how, to participants, anorexia may be a way of making and mapping the space of the present; not eating thereby emerges as a form of care that 'craft[s] more bearable ways of living with, or in, reality' (Mol 2008: 53). The virtual and actual foodwork of not eating, albeit ambivalently, mediates how participants encounter the worlds around them; it processually reproduces an illness that offers a way to withdraw from, or interact with, these. Such a conceptualization of the illness as 'crafting' the present is contrasted in some accounts with the uncertainty signified by the future. As Elisa put it, 'you don't quite know what the future holds' and, to her, this emphasized anorexia's safety. Thus, if caring comprises 'persistent tinkering in a world full of complex ambivalence and shifting tensions' (Mol et al. 2010b: 14), anorexia offers a way of caring for the self that navigates tensions; or, as Leila put it, 'anorexia looks after you'.

This sense of self-care through anorexia clearly diverges from the clinic's conceptualization of the illness. But there are also overlaps not only between ways of caring but also between how the clinic and participants envision the object of care. In the EDU the so-called 'authentic self' was at once the receiver and also goal of care, which positioned it within two temporalities at once. Here, as anorexia itself emerges as a modality of care, the self is cared for in the space of the present moment but in a way that may not offer any other temporality. Caring through not eating performs stasis rather than teleology, with all the ambiguity that 'stasis' suggests.

There is a precariousness to anorexia as a modality of self-care; its safe space is potentially consuming. Josie illustrated this in her interview by saying, 'I felt like I wasn't existing'. This slippage from a space of selfhood to one of effacement was also described by Lacey, who said the process from one to the other was 'like rolling down a slope'. Yet, despite the distress expressed at this sense of a loss of agency to, and sometimes betrayal by, anorexia, participants do not always wish to give up this particular modality of self-care; rather, their narratives evince an accommodation to the ways in which caring may be a deeply painful activity. This was clear in Hadia's interview when she recounted how she would sometimes sit and just, as she put it, 'be alone with anorexia'; she described feeling 'safe' and 'okay' in this space. But, Hadia also described how she would sometimes feel her anorexia becoming too strong, too entrapping in a way that 'pushed [her] out'. Yet, instead of this statement signifying a wholesale alignment with clinical conceptualizations, within it diverging paradigms touch edges before quickly parting ways. In order to care for herself within this entrapment, Hadia described working harder at her foodwork to processually reproduce the space of her illness and align herself with(in) it.

It was arguably therefore her experience of anorexia's narrowing of possibility that led Hadia to continually re-invent it as '[her] space'. In this, she illustrates that 'people make-do with what they have' (de Certeau 1984: 18), whilst also showing that anorexia as a mode of self-care could be regarded, following Plato, as a 'pharmakon' (2005; Derrida 2004); it is not only both remedy and poison at once but, importantly, remedy for its own poison. Evincing the doubledness encapsulated by the preposition 'through', self-care through anorexia sees anorexia as at once a vector of caring but also as something that is difficult to live through. These become enfolded as participants like Hadia work harder to catch up with anorexia so that it may continue to 'look after' them. The illness is thus a way 'to live with what would otherwise be unendurable' (Fischer 2007: 423) where the unendurable may be at once cause and effect.

Therefore, care-full dynamics of ordering and producing the everyday through the foodwork of not eating have been seen to enable a particular selfhood to emerge, albeit painfully and precariously, within and through anorexia. This, however, does not simply constitute a reversal of the clinic's paradigm of selfhood as in opposition to anorexia. Rather, the processual mapping of the present in participants' discussions points to an imagining of selfhood that is less bounded. Although conceptualizations of anorexia as skin and space seem de-relational, there is a complex sociality to many participants' narratives. Returning to Corin's metaphor of 'psychic skin' (2007: 283) illuminates this sense of connection as well as disconnection. As Michel Serres reminds us, skin is porous as 'in it, through it, with it, the world and my body touch each other' (2008: 80). Therefore, extending the existing sense of anorexia as that which maps encounters between inner and outer worlds, the final section will now explore a more relational ordering enacted by participants through the careful sociality of foodwork. If, in rematerializing the self through the body, the clinic performed care in a paradoxically dual and yet embodied way, in this discussion of anorexia *as* care the body has hovered at the periphery of the page, seemingly unrelated to anorexia or food. By now turning to explore how not eating cares for Others, troubled and troubling bodily materiality is brought finally into analysis.

Careful Sociality: (Not) Eating (and) Others

In her interview Rashida described how she had begun to self-starve after her father had been hospitalized for a terminal illness. She poignantly recounted having watched him 'shrinking away' and feeling that if she could 'just eat less than him', so that he would never become smaller than her, 'things would be okay'. Likewise, Elisa said of her sister's hospitalization when they were children:

> What I really remember hating when she was ill is seeing everyone else at school and all of her friends and all of my friends carrying on as normally and being healthy and laughing with each other and I really hated that because, you know, my sister was in hospital, it was like the end of my world, um, and I think I want, I wanted that to be marked and almost by punishing myself and by making things bad for me I was marking that and almost not putting myself in the same boat as her but giving myself something, something bad because I would have preferred it was me to be ill. (Elisa, outpatient, 2014)

Both Rashida and Elisa's accounts echo the discussions above of not eating as a modality of gaining control, particularly in emotionally distressing situations. Yet, they also evince the painful partiality of such control, as not eating may successfully map and maintain the space forged inside anorexia but is powerless beyond this. We might therefore be tempted to suggest that here we are confronted with the limits of conceptualizing – or even, experiencing – anorexia as caring. Yet reflecting again on not eating as active foodwork takes us beyond this to illuminate the place of emotional labour in this discussion; this elucidates how food, and its lack, are set to work here in a way that performs caring about Others.

In contrast to explorations of the caring implicit in commensality (see Carsten 1997), Rashida and Elisa's narratives frame the sharing of a lack of food as engendering threads of care between bodies and persons. If care is at once 'both a practice and a disposition' (Tronto 1993: 104) and the last section's discussion of self-care explored practices, care emerges here as an embodied disposition. In their felt powerlessness to care for their family members in any other way – to map the future or indeed present for their loved ones – Rashida and Elisa entangle their bodies into a performance of care, enacting a mimetic alignment. Elisa's words that she 'would have preferred it was [her] to be ill' frame her not eating as a 'somatic mode of attention' (Csordas 1993). That this may be at once 'attentive'

(Fisher and Tronto 1990) and yet not necessarily fully agential resonates through Elisa's words above, and elucidates that not eating may be a way caring *about* in the face of an inability to care *for.*

Although Rashida and Elisa's performances of care are embedded in the intimacies of familial relations, a similar mimetic alignment of suffering bodies, but across geographical distances, occurs in other participants' narratives of not eating. Some described how they had been chastized as children for not finishing the food on their plates with variations on the line 'think of the starving children'. They related this to a need to not consume 'too much', which was enacted through anorexia. Similarly, in her interview, Juno likened her not eating to the sponsored 24-hour famine established by the charity Vision UK in which participants raise money to aid victims of famine. Recent work has illuminated how eating is an act that engenders webs of sociality between eating bodies across spatial and temporal distances (Abbots and Lavis 2013). This has extended discussions of commensality to explore food as a substance that travels across distances, be those affective, material or both. Here Juno's words instead evince the sociality of shared absence; not eating mobilizes caring as an engagement with Others that seeks to 'maintain' or 'repair' the world (Tronto 1993: 102-3). It signifies an attentiveness forged through 'recognizing the needs of those around us' (ibid.: 127). It was Milla who most deeply expressed this during her interview; she described her anorexia as both 'an illness' and also 'a sort of testimony to the wrongness of the world'. In so doing, she referred to the philosophy of Simone Weil. It was Weil herself who wrote about attention that it 'consists in suspending thought, leaving it available, empty, and ready to be entered by its object' (Weil in Little 1988: 130). As such, together, 'testimony' and 'attention' articulate a sense of self-suspension that navigates between anorexia as self-protection and self-loss, whilst also intertwining these with the care of Others. Milla recounted how she was told she was 'too global' by staff in the EDU who felt she should 'focus on [her]self':

> I know I've been told over and over again 'your, your protest won't stop exploitation in the third world just because you know, you boycott coca cola it isn't going to stop them cutting down the rainforests' … . Erm and, 'what do you think the starving people would say if they saw you doing this to yourself?' All this stuff. Of course I know, of course I know. (Milla, inpatient, 2008)

It is perhaps as anorexia compromises conditions of possibility in the mingled protection and engulfment, seen above, that caring for Others offers a way of being oneself through the alternative becoming of mimesis. As such, linking one's self-starvation to other suffering bodies across geographical distances also reinforces a particular modality of self-production. It allows anorexia to be reinforced by the body of an imagined Other. The illness thereby becomes, at once, legitimized and moralized.

Scholars have previously explored anorexia in relation to cultural discourses of morality, arguing that 'anorexics [are] misguided moralists' (O'Connor and Van

Esterik 2008: 7). It has been suggested that eating disorders 'are the symptoms of ordinary morality, which is just being taken seriously – or more seriously than usual' (Giordano 2005: 8-9). Yet, with a few exceptions (see Gooldin 2008; Warin 2010), such discussions have tended to focus on anorexia's intersections with the wider cultural valuing of 'purity' and 'lightness' (Giordano 2005: 127) in a Euro-American context. Here instead it is food itself (and its lack), rather than the secondary effect of this on bodies, that emerges as a 'moral choice' (Coveney 1999: 33). As self-starvation maps nascent forms of careful sociality, it becomes 'an attempt to meet the other morally' (Noddings 2013: 707). This intersects with wider enactments of ethically concerned consumption (see Miele and Evans 2010) whilst also framing not eating as 'a moral achievement' (Tronto 1993: 127).

Yet, drawing on a moral framework in this way is also performative; it serves not only to mime and mediate Others but also produce them, mapping other bodies and other hungers over those of participants. As such not eating as a somatic modality of attending to the suffering of Others enacts a complex interplay of visibility and invisibility. We saw this in the somatic echoing of her father's illness in Rashida's narrative, above, as her not eating sought to nourish him by effacing her. Moreover, in this wider discussion of care in a global context, caring through not eating simultaneously forges links between bodies based on suffering, whilst also recognizing – or, perhaps, feeling – *only* the suffering of the Other's body. This gains a hyper-visibility whilst that of participants is maintained as peripheral. The doubledness and dualism in this is elucidated by turning to one participant, Michelle's, slippers.

'What can one say, I ask, about a slipper?' says Michel Serres (2008: 64). In the EDU many things were asked and uttered about Michelle's slippers. These were old, worn and not a little battered; her toe came through the end of one and the stripes had faded to grey. Staff often tried to convince Michelle to buy a new pair of slippers, drawing her attention to their visual appearance, which they described as 'uncared for'. To staff, thus, keeping these slippers was indicative of a wider lack of self-care. By delinking Michelle's slippers from anything but her body and her anorexia through this paradigm of self-care, the clinic thereby bound these together, as we saw above. Yet, Michelle felt that her slippers 'would do' as to replace them when they still 'worked as slippers', as she put it, would be 'wasteful'. To Michelle her slippers were entangled with her wider ethic of care as 'not consuming too much'. Michelle justified keeping her slippers by saying:

> The way society is now it just seems so complex and in terms of consumerism …
> there's this constant effort to produce a new variety or just something different.
> Or just, 'new extra this' – even cornflakes, you know, 'extra crunchy' with 'extra
> added this' … . 'added whatever', something that people think might be good
> for their health or improve their teeth of whatever … . Or types of teabags! It's
> just ridiculous the amount of choice. And there is just such a lot of waste and
> it creates, whether it's about food or anything, it creates an attitude that it's ok.

> But the amount of waste we produce is just ridiculous and it's actually shameful
> I think. Some people elsewhere would do anything for the minutest thing we
> throw away. (Michelle, inpatient, 2008)

Thus, to conceptualize Michelle's footwear only as metonymic of a lack of self-care enacted through not eating would privilege the visual narrative of both her slippers and her body over her voice. This would perhaps be care-less rather than care-full. Yet, the staff's discussions of Michelle's slippers have also highlighted a tension between embodiment and disembodiment that has resonated throughout this discussion of careful sociality. On the one hand, it has become clear that anorexia is about far more than a quest for corporeal emaciation; complex, relational and intimate practices of caring have shown the illness to be embodied and yet not *about* the body as a visual entity. As, at once, a profoundly 'somatic mode of attention' (Csordas 1993) to Others that forges affective links through bodies and their suffering, anorexia has also paradoxically emerged as something that effaces the body and enacts dualism. As not eating *as* self-care and careful sociality are contrasted to the clinic's vision of a lack of self-care within anorexia, competing paradigms of care not only frame bodily materialities in diverging ways but also 'interfere' (Haraway 2008) with these. Bodies become caught up in practices of caring for self and Others through food in ways that engender moments of encounter between anorexic ways of caring and those of the clinic.

In her interview Eva described the effects starvation had on her body; she recounted bones so sharp that when she turned over in bed she felt them scratching against her skin from within and described how her hair had fallen out and her skin dried to flakes. Before entering the EDU she had been frightened that she was about to go blind because her vision was so blurred. Here the somatic vulnerability of Eva's suffering body does seem, in line with the clinic's claims, to disrupt the caring performed by anorexia. Indeed, Tronto argues that 'in order to recognize the needs of others, one must first be attentive to one's own needs for care' (1993: 131). Here then, as in Michelle's slippers, caring for Others and self would seem to be difficult to align (see also Abbots, this volume). Yet, Eva said of this, 'anorexia's got nothing to do with my body. The physical bit's just a symptom of my mind'. In this simultaneous foregrounding of bodily suffering and yet repudiating of the body as 'important' to anorexia, lived corporeal materiality is re-framed as outside the relationship – the careful sociality, perhaps – between anorexia and self. This disallows embodied suffering to disrupt caring. Echoing Hadia's reconfigurations in relation to a felt loss of agency to anorexia above, here self-care and careful sociality are enfolded and, once again, placed beyond the painful as well as quantifiable perimetres of the body.

This delinking of body and self importantly also demonstrates how diverging ways of caring *about*, *for*, *through* and *within* anorexia, seen throughout this chapter, converge. This is because it allows Eva to engage in clinical treatment, seeking care for her bodily suffering whilst also holding onto anorexia and its ways of caring. She described feeling 'grateful' that the clinic had enforced her eating and thereby 'taken away the pain, but not anorexia'. We see, thus, how within the intimacies of bodily depths, diverging paradigms and scales of care co-exist and that caring perhaps always entails negotiation of co-existing as well as competing 'goods' (see Mol et al. 2010a). Eva allows herself to be cared for in a way that she feels to maintain her anorexia *and* selfhood. That this permits the illness to continue mapping the space of the present in ways that care for Eva warrants recognition as we listen to her narrative. Yet at the same time it perhaps also suggests that anorexia's 'careful sociality' may be, most of all, with itself.

Conclusion

It is viscerally clear why, in anorexia, 'the story of illness that trumps all others' (Frank 1997: 5) is the clinical. Yet, this chapter has sought to show that there are other stories that need attending to. For both the clinic, and individuals with anorexia, not eating keeps the illness present. Yet what is kept present, and indeed effaced, diverges. To the clinic anorexia signifies a lack; the present is effaced by illness so that clinical care is both of – and has as its goal the recovery of – the 'authentic self'. Through a food-as-medicine paradigm, eating becomes a linear modality of rematerializing this self, envisaged as lost through self-starvation. In contrast, to some individuals with anorexia the illness offers a way of living through the present; this is forged and mapped by, but also ambivalently contained within, anorexia. In these narratives, anorexia and self cannot be distinguished so neatly, as the illness offers a space of and for selfhood whilst also performing care about and for (imagined) Others. In the introduction, I called on an idea of bracketing to allow recognition of the clinical realities of anorexia whilst opening up a space in which to explore beyond these. As the chapter has unfurled, we have seen how these are also in tension in the lives of participants; illness and selves, bodies and pain, eating and caring, are all divergently and procesually positioned and bracketed in relation to one another. In particular, the materialities of foods and bodies have shifted in and out of view as ways of caring have engendered interplays of visibility and invisibility. Alongside this troubled and troubling materiality, it is perhaps both the distress and intermittent loss of agency in participants' lived experiences of anorexia that most problematizes an idea of the illness as care. Yet, it is also both of these that underpin its importance; caring is cyclical as care of the self necessarily instigates caring for anorexia so that it may continue to 'look after you'. Thus, this chapter has perhaps most shown that caring about individuals with anorexia depends 'to an important extent, on one's sense of empathy and compassion for a person's suffering' (2005: 261) as well, perhaps, on listening. By tracing along some of the sharper edges of both eating and caring, the discussion has sought to forge understandings of how care, food and anorexia are all lived and felt, resisted and reconfigured, in ways that disrupt but also 'matter' the intimacies of individual bodies, selves and everyday lives.

Acknowledgements

I should like to express my gratitude to the many individuals who have shared their stories with me during the course of this research and, in particular, I would like to remember J.T.

This chapter has drawn on two studies: The first (2007-2008 data) was my PhD, undertaken in the Anthropology Department at Goldsmiths, University of London. I thank my supervisors there, Simon Cohn and Catherine Alexander. This was funded by an Economic and Social Research Council studentship and received NHS ethical approval. The second study (2013-2014 data) is taking place at the University of Birmingham and I acknowledge my collaborators there: Newman Leung, Charlotte Connor, Max Birchwood, Sunita Channa and Colin Palmer. The study is funded by the NIHR Collaboration for Leadership in Applied Health Research (CLAHRC) and it received NHS ethical approval. The views expressed in this chapter are those of the author and not necessarily those of the NHS, CLAHRC or the Department of Health.

References

Abbots, E-J. and Lavis, A. (eds) 2013. *Why We Eat, How We Eat: Contemporary Encounters between Foods and Bodies*. Farnham: Ashgate.

American Psychiatric Association. 2013. *Diagnostic and Statistical Manual of Mental Disorders*. 5th Edition. Arlington, VA: American Psychiatric Publishing.

Barnes, M. 2012. *Care in Everyday Life: An Ethic of Care in Practice*. Bristol: Policy Press.

Berg, M. and Mol, A. (eds) 1998. *Differences in Medicine: Unravelling Practices, Techniques and Bodies*. Durham and London: Duke University Press.

Biehl, J.O. and Locke, P. 2010. Deleuze and the anthropology of becoming. *Current Anthropology*, 51(3), 317-51.

Bogle, I. 2000 (May). *Eating Disorders, Body Image and the Media*. London: British Medical Association Board of Science and Education Pamphlet.

Bruch, H. 1974. *Eating Disorders: Obesity, Anorexia and the Person Within*. London: Routledge and Kegan Paul.

Carsten, J. 1997. *The Heat of the Hearth: The Process of Kinship in a Malay Fishing Community*. Oxford: Clarendon Press.

Corin, E. 2007. The 'Other' of culture in psychosis: The ex-centricity of the subject, in *Subjectivity: Ethnographic Investigations*, edited by J. Bieh, B. Good and A. Kleinman. Berkeley, CA: University of California Press, 273-314.

Coveney, J. 1999. *The Pleasure and Anxiety of Eating*. London: Routledge.

Csordas, Thomas. 1993. Somatic modes of attention. *Cultural Anthropology*, 8(2), 135-56.

de Certeau, M. 1984. *The Practice of Everyday Life*. Berkeley, CA and Los Angeles, CA: University of California Press.

Derrida, J. 2004. *Dissemination*. London and New York: Continuum.

Draper, H. 2000. Anorexia nervosa and respecting a refusal of life-prolonging therapy: A limited justification. *Bioethics*, 4(2), 120-33.

Eivors, A., Button, E., Warner, S. and Turner, K. 2003. Understanding the experience of drop-out from treatment for anorexia nervosa. *European Eating Disorders Review*, 11(2), 90-107.

Eli, K. 2014. Between difference and belonging: Configuring Self and Others in inpatient treatment for eating disorders. *PLoS ONE* 9(9)

Fischer, M.J. 2007. To live with what would otherwise be unendurable: Return(s) to subjectivities, in *Subjectivity: Ethnographic Investigations*, edited by J. Biehl, B. Good and A. Kleinman. Berkeley, CA: University of California Press, 423-46.

Fisher, B. and Tronto, J. 1990. Toward a feminist theory of caring, in *Circles of Care. Work and Identity in Women's Lives*, edited by E. Abel and M. Nelson. Albany, NY: State University of New York Press, 35-62.

Foucault, M. 2003. *The Birth of the Clinic: An Archaeology of Medical Perception*. London and New York: Routledge Classics.

Frank, A. 1997. *The Wounded Storyteller: Body, Illness and Ethics*. Chicago and London: University of Chicago Press.

Giordano, S. 2005. *Understanding Eating Disorders: Conceptual and Ethical Issues in the Treatment of Anorexia and Bulimia Nervosa*. Oxford: Oxford University Press.

Gooldin, S. 2008. Being anorexic: Hunger, subjectivity and embodied morality. *Medical Anthropology Quarterly*, 22(3), 274-96.

Gremilllion, H. 2003. Feeding Anorexia: Gender and Power at the Treatment Centre. Durham and London: Duke University Press.

Griffiths, R. and Russell, J. 1998. Compulsory treatment of anorexia nervosa patients, in *Treating Eating Disorders: Ethical, Legal and Personal Issues*, edited by W. Vandereycken and P. Beaumont. London: The Athlone Press, 127-50.

Harbers, H., Mol, A. and Stollmeyer. 2002. Food matters: Arguments for an ethnography of daily care. *Theory, Culture and Society*, 19(5-6), 207-26.

Haraway, D. 2008. Otherwordly conversations, terran topics, local terms, in *Material Feminisms*, edited by S. Alaimo and S. Hekman. Bloomington, IN: Indiana University Press, 157-87.

Heaven, B., Bamford, C., May, C. and Moynihan, P. 2013. Food work and feeding assistance on hospital wards. *Sociology of Health & Illness*, 35(4), 628-42.

Held, V. 2006. *The Ethics of Care: Personal, Political, and Global*. Oxford: Oxford University Press.

Heuts, F. and Mol, A. 2013. What is a good tomato? A case of valuing in practice. *Valuation Studies*, 1(2) 125-46.

Jackson, M. 2002. Familiar and foreign bodies: A phenomenological exploration of the human-technology interface. *Journal of the Royal Anthropological Institute (New Series)*, 8(2), 333-46.

Lavis, A. 2013. The substance of absence: Exploring eating and anorexia, in *Why We Eat, How We Eat: Contemporary Encounters Between Foods and Bodies*, edited by E-J. Abbots and A. Lavis. Farnham: Ashgate, 35-52.

Lavis, A. 2014. Engrossing encounters: Materialities and metaphors of fat in the lived experiences of individuals with anorexia, in *Fat: Culture and Materiality*, edited by C. Forth and A Leitch. London: Bloomsbury, 91-108.

Little, P. 1988. *Simone Weil: Waiting on Truth.* New York: St Martin's Press.

Long, S., Wallis, D.J., Leung, N., Arcelus, J. and Meyer, C. 2012. Mealtimes on eating disorder wards: A two-study investigation. *International Journal of Eating Disorders*, 45(2), 241-6.

Matusek, J and Wright, M.O. 2010. Ethical dilemmas in treating clients with eating disorders: A review and application of an integrative ethical decision-making model. *European Eating Disorders Review*, 18(6), 434-52.

Melamed, Y., Mester, R., Margolin, J. and Kallan, M. 2003. Involuntary treatment of anorexia nervosa. *International Journal of Law and Psychiatry*, 26(6), 617-26.

Miele, M. and Evans, A.B. 2010. When foods become animals: Ruminations on ethics and responsibility in care-full practices of consumption. *Ethics Place and Environment*, 13(2), 171-90.

Mol, A. 2008. *The Logic of Care: Health and the Problem of Patient Choice.* London: Routledge.

Mol, A. 2010. Care and its values: Good food in the nursing home, in *Care in Practice: On Tinkering in Clinics, Homes and Farms*, edited by A. Mol et al. New London: Transaction Publishers, 215-34.

Mol, A. 2012. Mind your plate! The ontonorms of Dutch dieting. *Social Studies of Science*, 0(0), 1-18.

Mol, A., Moser, I. and Pols, J. (eds) 2010a. *Care in Practice: On Tinkering in Clinics, Homes and Farms.* New London: Transaction Publishers.

Mol, A, Moser, I. and Pols, J. 2010b. Care: Putting practice into theory, in *Care in Practice: On Tinkering in Clinics, Homes and Farms*, edited by A. Mol et al. New London: Transaction Publishers, 7-26.

NICE 2004. *Eating Disorders: Core Interventions in the Treatment and Management of Anorexia Nervosa, Bulimia Nervosa and Related Eating Disorders, National Collaborating Centre for Mental Health.* London: The British Psychological Society and Gaskell.

Noddings, N. 2013. An ethic of caring, in *Ethical Theory: An Anthology*, edited by R. Shafer-Landau. Oxford: Wiley Blackwell, 699-712.

O'Connor, R.A. and Van Esterik, P. 2008. De-medicalizing anorexia: A new cultural brokering. *Anthropology Today*, 24(5), 6-9.

Palmer, B. 2014. *Helping People with Eating Disorders: A Clinical Guide to Assessment and Treatment (second edition).* Chichester: Wiley Blackwell.

Pierson, C.A. 1999. Ethnomethodological analysis of account of feeding demented residents in long-term care. *Journal of Nursing Scholarship*, 31(2), 127-31.

Plato 2005. *Phaedrus.* London: Penguin Classics.

Pols, J. 2013. Washing the patient: Dignity and aesthetic values in nursing care. *Nursing Philosophy*, 14(3), 186-200.

Powers, P.S and Cloak, N.L 2013. Failure to feed patients with anorexia nervosa and other perils and perplexities in the medical care of eating disorder patients. *Eating Disorders: The Journal of Treatment & Prevention*, 21(1), 81-9.

Serres, M. 2008. *The Five Senses: A Philosophy of Mingled Bodies (I)*. London: New York, Continuum.

Tan, J. 2003. The Anorexia Talking? *The Lancet*, 362(9391), 1246.

Tan, J. and Hope, T. 2008. Treatment refusal in anorexia nervosa: A challenge to current concepts of capacity, in *Empirical Ethics in Psychiatry*, edited by G. Widdershoven, J. McMillan, T. Hope and L. Van Der Scheer. Oxford: Oxford University Press, 187-210.

Tan, J., Stewart, A., Fitzpatrick, R. and Hope, T. 2010. Attitudes of patients with anorexia nervosa to compulsory treatment and coercion. *International Journal of Law and Psychiatry*, 33(1), 13-19.

Tronto, J. 1993. *Moral Boundaries: A Political Argument for an Ethic of Care*. London: Routledge.

Treasure, J., Smith, G. and Crane, A. 2007. *Skills-based Learning for Caring for a Loved One with an Eating Disorder: The New Maudsley Method*. London: Routledge.

Treasure, J. and Schmidt, U. 2005, Treatment overview, in *The Essential Handbook of Eating Disorders*, edited by J. Treasure, U. Schmidt and E. Van Furth. Chichester: Wiley, 91-102.

Treasure, J. and Ward, A. 1997. A practical guide to the use of motivational interviewing in anorexia nervosa. *European Eating Disorders Review*, 5(2), 102-14.

Twigg, J. 2002. *Bathing: The Body and Community Care*. London: Routledge.

Twigg, J. 2006. *The Body in Health and Social Care*. Basingstoke: Palgrave Macmillan.

Ungerson, C. 1983. Why do women care?, in *A Labour of Love: Women, Work and Caring*, edited by J. Finch and D. Groves. London: Routledge and Kegan Paul, 41-9.

Vitousek, K.B. 2005. Alienating patients from the "Anorexic Self": Externalizing and related strategies. London: Seventh International Conference on Eating Disorders.

Warin, M. 2010. *Abject Relations: Everyday Worlds of Anorexia*. New Brunswick, NJ and London: Rutgers University Press.

Willems, D. 1998. Inhaling drugs and making worlds: A proliferation of lungs and asthmas, in *Differences in Medicine: Unravelling Practices, Techniques, and Bodies*, edited by M. Berg and A. Mol. Durham, NC: Duke University Press, 105-18.

Williams, P.M., Goodie, J. and Motsinger, C.D. 2008. Treating eating disorders in primary care. *American Family Physician*, 77, 187-95.

Chapter 5

The Sweetness of Care: Biographies, Bodies and Place

Tanya Zivkovic, Megan Warin, Vivienne Moore,
Paul Ward and Michelle Jones

Introduction

> Lyn is an overweight mother of five children. She is in a domestically violent
> relationship with a man on the methadone program and she has a heart condition.
> Since losing over $100 a week from her government benefits, she can no longer
> run a car, safely transport her kids to school or pay for their uniforms. One of
> her children has Asperger Syndrome. While doing her food shopping she buys
> a cheap cake mix and tells me her body 'craves sweet things'. She said 'I really
> try to be healthy and to not eat crap but you know I've got a sweet tooth and
> sometimes when things really get under my skin, I'll think to myself 'go on then,
> have some chocolate'.

We begin with this vignette to illustrate how sweetness intersects bodies, place and
care at a time when Australia is running its largest obesity prevention program –
OPAL (Obesity Prevention and Lifestyle). We conducted ethnographic research
over twenty-three months with socially disadvantaged families in Adelaide, South
Australia (August 2012 – July 2014). Our aim was to explore how families in
this community respond to, negotiate and/or resist 'healthy lifestyle' messages
when healthy living guidelines may present a 'disconnect' with the adversities of
everyday life (Lindsay 2010). Health promotion initiatives urge this population
to care for their own bodies and those of their families through a range of social
marketing messages, including reducing sugar intake.

Tracing the historical development of nutritional science from its moral
Christian beginnings, Coveney (1999) reveals how foods that impart flavour and
pleasure (e.g. sugar, fat, salt) have been restricted (and constructed as 'sinful')
in dietary discourse. In accordance with this moral weight attributed to food,
not all sugars are created equal. Australian (and international) dietary guidelines
encourage populations to 'Eat more fruit and vegetables' *and* to 'Eat less sugar',
taking for granted distinctions between foods that contain 'natural' sugars – and
are viewed as 'good' – and the 'harmful', 'added' sugars of 'bad' processed foods
and confectionary. Lyn has adopted this advice, categorising refined sugars as
'sometimes foods'. Yet, whilst she constantly abstains from the ingredients that

she associates with pleasure and taste, eating sweet things in the form of refined sugars also provides her with the 'small pleasures' she needs to care for herself and to cope with the adverse circumstances of her everyday life. As such, Lyn's words show that, in places where hardship can 'get under one's skin', people may care for themselves and others in ways that counter dominant healthy eating messages.

Nutritional scientists assert that a preference for sweet tastes appears to be part of our 'basic biology' (Mennella and Ventura 2010). Before birth, a sweet taste prompts increased swallowing of amniotic fluid and in early infancy, sweet solutions elicit a variety of responses that are positive or hedonic (such as lip smacking or finger sucking). Breast milk is sweet as it is high in lactose or milk sugar (Hall 1979) as are commercial infant formulae based on the composition of breast milk. From very early in life, it is therefore suggested, we learn to associate sweetness with feeding and comfort. While this illustrates the bodily materialities of sugar (in utero, early life and taste receptors on a tongue), its reception is culturally shaped and embedded. In his classic study, Mintz (1985) shows how the taste of sweetness (associated particularly with sugar production) had a distinctive history that altered not only diets in the West, but equally impacted notions of time, gender and class, as well as senses of self – especially in relation to family, community and labour. Extending Mintz's groundbreaking work on the political economy of sweetness, other anthropologists using sensory approaches (Seremetakis 1994; Stoller 1989) have similarly shown how sugar is entangled in social relations (Cowan 1990, 1991; Warin and Dennis 2005). For example, Cowan (1991) and Warin and Dennis (2005) have demonstrated how sweetness and the senses are deeply entwined, in that apparently natural or taken-for-granted practices of sensorily encountering sugar (e.g. eating it, tasting it, smelling it, seeing it) are invested with meaning, emotion, memory, and value. Fragrant hot black tea sucked through lumps of hard Persian sugar connect otherwise distant sites of Iranian homes, sociality, past and present (Warin and Dennis 2005). The ingestion of locally produced fruit-flavored liqueur in Greece, served in 'a richly adorned thin-stemmed glass [of] silver or crystal' enables Sohoian 'girls and women [to] literally produce themselves as properly feminine persons' (Cowan 1990: 65-6).

As recent research on care and food has elucidated, it is 'not only the *substance*, food,' that has value (e.g. nutritional value) but 'the *practice*, eating, is at least as important' (Mol 2010: 217, emphasis in original). As Mol argues, the ambience, aesthetics and relationality of food not only shape or constrain the practice of eating but also the nutritional value, the substance consumed. In this chapter we highlight how sugar as chemical substance and sweetness as relational experience are intimately, and at times uneasily, linked in the lives and lounge-rooms of our participants. We approach sweetening as a way to comfort and connect through momentary pleasures involving those 'bad' sugars which are constructed as sinful (ascetically and nutritionally) in health discourse. We propose that sweetening is a useful conceptual category for thinking through the discordance between public health understandings of sugar and how ethnography reveals local contingencies of care through sweetness.

While sweetening is widespread and may operate in all of our lives, this chapter explores how it is enacted as a practice of care in Playford, a place of social disadvantage. Following Mol's idea of care as a process of 'tinkering' (2010; Mol et al. 2010a) that involves 'crafting more bearable ways of living with, or in, reality' (Mol 2008: 53), we show how care is configured in the context of food, eating and disadvantage. Sweetness, we argue, emerges as a strategy of caring (for oneself and for others) practised by low-income families to negotiate social hierarchies and relations, and sweeten circumstances that have gone sour. Families thereby reclaim the meanings of sugar beyond a nutritional discourse of 'dietary sugar' and 'sweetness' permeates everyday language as people are described as 'sweetie' or 'honey', things are 'sweet' and circumstances become palatable. As such, we view sweetness *as* a practice of care.

It is therefore the everyday forms of resistance and the reclaiming of both care and sugar from public health discourse that we develop in this chapter through the concept of 'sweetening'. Contrasting discourses and practices of care are contested in the meanings of sweet foods. Anthropologists and care theorists highlight the political malleability of 'care': how care can be used to support different political agendas (Tronto 1993) that inform cultural imaginings of food and eating (cf. Mol 2010). Care, as it is employed in healthcare or healthy lifestyle programs, is embedded in culturally-entrenched understandings of what is morally 'right' and what is 'good', both for bodies and for society (Barnes 2012; Held 2006). Eating 'good' food and performing the 'right' activities are valued by health interventions such as OPAL as ways to educate and support families to care for themselves and for others (by eating and sharing these 'right' foods). 'Good intentions' are implicit in these understandings of care (Mol et al. 2010a: 12) and are taken-for-granted in obesity prevention strategies. As this chapter demonstrates however, this caring that aims to stop people from eating and drinking the substances that are cheap, plentiful and tasty misses its mark because asking people to refrain from one of the few things that makes them feel good, feels uncaring. These tensions between how care is understood and experienced differently need to be foregrounded to account for the effects of socio-economic inequities on bodies.

Margaret Lock's concept of 'local biologies' (1993) has challenged the notion of a universal, 'natural' and readily standardizable body, and foregrounded bodies as at once both socio-political and material, whilst also being products of individual lived experiences in specific environmental, historical, and socio-political contexts. We draw on this concept of local biologies to trace the ways in which sugar and sweetness are 'craved' by hungry bodies, and used in the everyday negotiation of social relations to enact care. In exploring how bodies, place and care meet in a semiotics and embodied politics of 'sweetness', we attend to the body as 'embedded' in both material and social processes and circumstances (Niewöhner 2011), tracing the intimate entanglement of physiological responses to the taste of sugar and the sweetening of social relations. By considering the frictions and complexities that come together in families' consumption of sweet foods, this chapter dislodges care from its associations with 'good intent' (Mol et al. 2010b) and critically examines how care *through* sweetening is entangled with, and shapes, both bodies and lives.

Challenges to Care in a Place of Poor Health

Playford is a place that has pockets of *Deep and Persistent Disadvantage* (McLachlan et al. 2013) and is rated as one of the most disadvantaged areas in Australia (Hordacre et al. 2013). A third of households live in poverty and there is a high incidence of unemployment and sole parent families (ibid.: 2013). As comparative studies in low and high-income areas of Adelaide show, low-income families spend a higher proportion of their income on food and this is constrained by other household expenses (including the rising costs in housing and utilities), leading to a greater prevalence of 'food stress' (Ward et al. 2013; Wong et al. 2011). The majority of families in our study conveyed that healthy foods were outside their purchasing power and, as a result, cheaper foods, which tend to be higher in fat or sugar, became more enticing out of a 'taste of necessity' (Bourdieu 1984: 178).

There is a significant body of research that has explored relationships between place and health inequalities (Popay et al. 2003; Pearce et al. 2012) and it is well established that people living in disadvantaged areas experience poorer health (Putland et al. 2011). A negative gradient between SES and health is typical of the relationship between class and most measures of health risk or outcome (Commission on Social Determinants of Health 2008). This is apparent in an analysis of 2010 Australian Bureau of Statistics data commissioned by the Australian federal government, which found that almost a quarter of adults living in the City of Playford reported their health as 'poor' (24 percent compared to 17 percent in the Adelaide metropolitan area) (Hordacre et al. 2013). In a paper titled the *Imperfect bodies of the poor*, social historian Peel (2004), who grew up in Playford, points to how poverty is inscribed in place *and* also in bodies: in crooked backs, missing teeth, and prematurely aged, frail or obese bodies. These entanglements of place and poverty in the local biologies of bodies is evident in Playford, where obesity prevalence is high, with 70.7 percent of people self-reporting as overweight or obese according to standard BMI measures (The University of Adelaide 2014).

The OPAL program was initiated in twenty South Australian communities, including two in Playford. Identified using place-based strategies, selected geographical areas were marked as being 'in need' of obesity prevention and lifestyle change. Obesity is approached as a public health issue in which unhealthy eating and lack of physical activity present risk factors for chronic disease and OPAL was one of the first Australian programs to manage this 'risk' through partnerships with South Australian local governments and local businesses. Through cooperative partnerships with local businesses OPAL has increased the availability and sales of fresh fruit and vegetables and lean cuts of meat at one local supermarket and increased the sales of bottled water (by reducing its cost) instead of soft drinks at a local recreation centre. These efforts underscore taken-for-granted hierarchies of nutritional value, elevating the status of some sugars and displacing the value and accessibility of others.

In the OPAL programme, public health knowledge about added sugar is foregrounded by its 'empty' caloric character but not the satiating sensory and emotional dimensions that are experienced, and which are detailed in the following sections of this chapter.[1] In training sessions and promotional materials for 'healthy eating' the unseen quantities of dissolved sugar in products like breakfast cereals and fizzy drinks are visually displayed, and measured in teaspoon-equivalent cubes. Publically revealing sugar quantities becomes a way to educate people about the foods that are high in sugar, are not healthy and should be eaten, as per the Federal government's *Australian Dietary Guidelines* 'only sometimes and in small amounts' (National Health and Medical Research Council 2013: 10). The relevance of corporeal engagements with both the substance of sugar and the feeling it provokes is thus overlooked. In prioritizing nutritional information over sensory encounters with food (Hartwick et al. 2014), sugar is framed as a substance to be measured, and its consumption controlled. This portrait of harm ignores how disadvantage, poverty, sustained unemployment and precarious livelihoods impact on people's abilities to change 'lifestyle behaviours'. Participants live in cycles of financial and food scarcity, and many have learned to live thrifty lives.

Many participants admitted to skipping meals, particularly breakfast as a deliberate financial strategy to make their money and their food 'stretch', like John who in his early 40s lives on his Newstart Allowance. John admitted, 'Oh, I'll often skip breakfast. If I've got no money, I gotta get by the cheapest way I can'. The challenges to caring for oneself and for others in this context of poverty and poor health was expressed by Ben. Long-term unemployed, overweight and in poor health, Ben asserted that his work prospects were negligible. 'I've got a bad back, depression and anxiety. I'm on the methadone program and I've also got a heart problem. Who on earth is going to employ me?' Living in a household of eight people who are all reliant on welfare payments is a continual financial struggle for which his family had been referred by Centrelink, Australia's social security government welfare branch, for counselling:

> We were left with only $25 a fortnight for all eight of us to live on after all expenses had been paid, the rent, bills etcetera. If anything unexpected came up we would be in the shit house … Seriously though, how can we manage our finances without being in financial hardship when we're only left with $25 a fortnight for eight people?

---

1   In nutrition discourses the term 'empty calories' refers to food and drinks that supply energy but little or no nutrition.

The unequal distributions of power, money and resources encountered in the day-to-day lives of Ben and his family structure the location and quality of their housing; educational opportunities; access to public transport, and food and medical care. All are influential determinants of their health (Drewnowski 2012; Offer et al. 2012).

That 'inequality gets under the skin' to affect the functioning of bodies has been raised by epidemiologists Wilkinson and Pickett in their book on societal inequalities, *The Spirit Level* (2009), which describes how population health and negative emotions, such as stress and anxiety, are intricately tied to social position. Extending their argument, sociologists Peacock et al. analyse how people deploy 'collective imaginaries' as part of a repertoire of techniques for reconfiguring identities and resisting structural inequalities which 'get inside the body and impact on health' (2014: 390). Attending to an intertwining of bodies, place, and care reveals how social disadvantage enters the *interiority* of bodies; how, for example, housing and economic insecurities and addictions affect the physiology of nerves, blood flow to the heart and skeletal functioning through anxiety, angina and aching backs. These 'local biologies' (Lock 1993, 2013) of disadvantage are situational and they traverse bodily boundaries: whether it is medicating with methadone or sweetening social life through sugar consumption, substances and addictions act on social life in ways that go far beyond notions of being 'unhealthy' to bodies. It is in this context that we explore opportunistic eating and the physiological responses to hunger, articulating the entanglements of both biology and culture.

Writing from a psychological perspective, Bryant et al. (2007) refer to 'opportunistic eating' as disinhibition; 'a tendency towards over-eating and eating opportunistically in an obesogenic environment' (ibid.: 409). Importantly, their study also highlights how factors such as stress and disadvantage are associated with making fewer healthful food choices (ibid.: 411) and increased consumption, especially of sweet foods. These authors suggest that along with gender and shared environmental factors – what we would call *habitus* (Bourdieu 1977) – that there may be some associated biological reasons for these sweet food preferences. While outside the scope of this chapter, there is certainly cause to examine the ways in which hunger, economic insecurity and abundance of high-sugar and high-fat foods are implicated in terms of adipose tissue processes, metabolism and muscle physiology, increased brain activity and differing levels of hunger and satiety related peptides. Or as Landecker suggests, how 'things outside of the body are transformed into the biology of the body' (2011: 178). Psychological studies on the adaptive physiological responses to the external world, such as 'thrifty phenotypes' and 'disinhibition' (Bryant et al. 2007), speak to the entanglements of biology and culture. Anthropologically speaking, these local biologies are implicated in the competing paradigms of care that are embodied and negotiated in the everyday lives of research participants living in Playford.

Our findings suggest that it is essential to consider how social disadvantage creates conceptualizations of eating and care that are different from public health admonitions, and that sweetening difficult circumstances is important to pleasure, place and social relations. For our research participants in Playford, the negotiation of their position in the world involved responding to circumstances of disadvantage with and through their bodies, by caring through food for themselves and for others.

Care for the Self

Participants involved in our study describe knowing that sugar is deemed in clinical terms to be unhealthy, implicating its consumption in diabetes and weight gain, but this understanding exists alongside other multiple meanings. Sugar may be empty calories but it is not an empty category. Caring for oneself by eating sweet foods is associated in our participants' narratives with cravings, desires and their fulfilment, but also with unwanted weight gain and health problems. These contrasting and at times competing experiences of sugar consumption and its effects are apparent in the disclosure of an 18 year old participant, Sienna. Describing herself as 'skinny but a little pudgy', Sienna says that parts of her body are 'very flabby' and she conceals her arms and stomach, admitting that she never wears tee-shirts but is fond of sporting tight stockings or long socks under short skirts.

Sienna has a history of what she terms 'severe depression and anxiety' and reports being a 'fussy eater' since the age of four. Sienna is disgusted by the taste of vegetables; she dislikes most meats; salads make her shudder; she despises the smell of mushrooms; can't eat nuts; won't touch seafood; rarely eats bread; avoids spicy food; hates the taste of milk; abhors rice and doesn't eat eggs. In our first interview, Sienna revealed that her self-described 'fussiness' emerged after her parents' separation when she was around two and that it intensified in the course of a custody battle, after which her father moved interstate for a decade, an event which she described as 'still reeling from'. Sienna said, 'I had no control over my life except for what I could eat because of all the custody drama, you know, I didn't feel in control. So, I would pick what I ate. And it's just kind of stuck with me'. It is not only the avoidance of some foods that forms part of Sienna's coping strategy, learnt from an early age, for dealing with the vicissitudes of social life. Conversely the taste and provision of other foods are equally important, marking levels of social cohesion. When asked what she does to get by when stressful things happen, Sienna says she eats 'comfort foods'.

While pleasure is constrained in Sienna's household by physical illness and psychological distress, sweetness is gained through the consumption of 'junk food like chocolate, chips, anything your heart desires and craves at that moment, you know, soft drink ... because if you're stressed out, you kind of need something. I deserve this. This is going to help me. Usually, for me, it's comfort food'. While sweetening social life through sugary foods is a practice Sienna uses to comfort and care for herself, she also positions sugar as dangerous saying:

> Hey, I got to stop this 'cause if I keep doing this I'm gonna get *really* fat, and that's really bad ... because you know, the larger you are, the more chance that, you know, the higher chance of you developing diabetes or, you know, being overweight means there's a few years cut off your life, you know?

Sienna's knowledge about the harmful effects of sugar and fat does not instigate a change in her eating practices. Observing a higher prevalence of obesity in her neighbourhood, Sienna commented, 'everything is just really crap around here it's like you just want to comfort eat 'cause everything sucks, so yeah'. Consuming sugar holds multiple meanings that surpass nutritional factors. It can be an active agent in achieving moments of pleasure and comfort amidst bitter circumstances, and sweetness can be embodied and experienced as self-care in the consumption of sweet foods. Relishing comfort foods is also an act of resistance against public health imperative of healthy eating. Chocolates are sometimes squirreled away, hidden in Sienna's bedroom and eaten in secret. Enacted at night either in the privacy of her bedroom or with her mother in the living-room, 'comfort eating' is a way to candy-coat the stressors of day-to-day social life; the threat of violent neighbours, ubiquitous financial insecurity and the routine of performing social pleasantries in her poorly paid, part-time and precarious customer service job. To Sienna, people who 'come through my register and steal things' or who are 'just so rude' and neighbours who can become violent and who threaten 'to bash me with a metal pole' are part and parcel of living in the area. 'Everyone up here is so rude. And like in the city they're kind of snobby, but at least they're nice if you talk to them. Here it's like, 'I hate you because you looked at me funny!''

Sienna's statements echo with popular stereotypes about 'ferals' or 'bogans' who live north of Adelaide and she reveals how these stereotypes also become a resource for the disadvantaged, as people 'play up to' and leverage on these stereotypes for their own benefit.[2] Social scientists have long reflected on how the limited agency of subordinate classes to mobilize and upset social hierarchies can facilitate the proliferation of small-scale acts of resistance (such as petty theft) (de Certeau 1984; Scott 1985) and the regaining of symbolic power (Bourdieu 1984). Tactics used to subvert power relations can be seen amongst disadvantaged communities in Newcastle upon Tyne, in the UK, where a 'black market' trade in contraband 'junk' foods operates among disenfranchized students revealing resistance to healthy school lunches, which is documented in a film clip entitled *Bro, are you selling?* (Ahmed 2013; see also Truninger and Teixeira, this volume). In this era of health and lifestyle management, we propose that these 'weapons of the weak' (Scott 1985) be extended to other embodied activities. Sweetening, we argue, serves to highlight structured cleavages of (bio)power and is a strategy of resistance against public health regulations on eating that people living in Playford creatively perform.

---

2 'Feral' or 'bogan' are Australian terms that connote 'rough' working-class cultural identities, much like the 'chav' in the UK (Hollingworth and Williams 2009; Nayak 2006).

It is in relation to this daily grind of disadvantage that some families living in Playford pose a challenge to public health conceptualizations of sugar as mere 'empty calories', and reclaim the meanings of sweetness in their local worlds. Sugary foods, in places of locational poverty, can sweeten moments of discomfort and, as in the following case of Jude, provide an accessible way to 'tinker' (Mol et al. 2010b: 13) with one's body and emotions through sensory gratification and enacting care for oneself.

Jude was born to working class UK migrant parents struggling to make ends meet. She described her parents as 'heavy drinkers' and 'hard on her', recalling that they made her undertake the majority of household domestic tasks as a young girl. Being conceived out of an affair and living in a poor household were the two reasons Jude cited for her parents' attitude to her. At the age of 11 she was sent to live with a family friend in a bakery where she worked the night shift until the age of 16. With disrupted educational opportunities Jude married a man in her late teens who beat her severely. 'He was a real madman. He broke all my fingers. He slashed my face open', she said while lifting her chin to show me the scar. To stop the 'flashbacks' of the beatings (that occurred 30 years ago) Jude takes anti-depressants. She said, 'They stop me from remembering the things you don't want to remember'. When ten years into the marriage the abuse was inflicted onto their young son, Jude left her husband. Soon after however, she entered into another domestically violent marriage and had a second son. In the course of the two abusive relationships Jude habitually overate, often seeking pleasure from ice-cream. Reflecting on this period of her life Jude exclaimed: 'I was starting depression then because of what I was going through' and 'I was eating really bad … I did not care about my body or weight' which escalated to 140kg. Indulging in ice-cream enabled Jude to experience some pleasure during discomfort, which she explained as a strategy to 'survive in the moment the best way I could'.

This over-consumption of 'comfort foods' is no longer part of Jude's repertoire of techniques for coping with adversity. Now diabetic, and having had a gastrectomy to treat stomach cancer, she is unable to digest foods that are high in fat or sugar. By repositioning previous food practices as harmful, Jude described how her current ways of eating and preparing whole foods are informed by public health principles of healthy eating. She said, 'in a way I was abusing my own self but not realizing that's what I was doing'. As Jude's biographical narrative shows, sugar can lead to weight gain and be harmful to the body, but its consumption may also be a strategy, albeit not necessarily a conscious one, to attenuate unhappiness and disadvantage through material and gustatory pleasure. For Sienna and Jude eating sweet treats reveals tensions between contextual experiences of 'comfort eating' and the dietary discourses that construct high-sugar diets as careless eating. The practice of caring for the self by 'sweetening' social life can be biologically damaging and, at the same time, can enable 'survival', offering a taste of something pleasant during times of hardship.

In their work on the social aspects of dietary sugars, McLennan et al. (2014) link the seemingly contradictory meanings of sugar as both 'good' and 'bad' to the commodification and corporate branding of sugar products. Self-care through consuming products that are bad for health is part of a pervasive marketing strategy. Sugar is transformed into a commodity that is fetishized as imbued with elevated status or mood – including sexual arousal and climax 'for pleasure seekers' satisfied by Magnum ice-creams such as 'Lust' in the 'Seven Deadly Sins' range. Sugary products, their packaging and advertisements make possible an experience of luxury and happiness in an impoverished place. In the everyday advertising of popular chocolates, consumers of Cadbury chocolates are transported to 'Joyville' or invited by Fererro Rocher to 'share the secret of gold', while the purchase of Mars-owned Dove confers an experience that is 'silky smooth' and Bounty is filled with a 'taste of paradise'. These chocolates are frequently mentioned as desirable by participants such as Karen, a single mother of two, who buys blocks of Dove in large quantities when they are on special. These chocolates enable the imagining, however briefly, of a taste of luxury, rather than a 'taste of necessity' (Bourdieu 1984: 178).

Care for Others: Social Relations

While sweetness is often used and marketed towards care for the self, it is also critical in our care for others. Rewarding children with lollipops and ice-cream, demonstrating appreciation or adoration with a box of chocolates, and celebrating the progression of others' years with a birthday cake are culturally normative exchanges that sweeten social relations. This sweetening of social life is played out in the relationship between Sienna and her mother with whom she lives.

Ironically having chosen the pseudonym Candy, Sienna's mother described purchasing the foods that sweeten her daughter's moments of anxiety and depression. Candy's identity is intricately related to her position as a mother. Having moved out of her natal home at the age of 13, Candy enjoys being the caretaker and provider for her 18 year old daughter and also nurtures other young boarders who live in her home. Candy buys the foods she knows Sienna will eat and drink, usually sweet tasting soft drinks, processed pasta sachets and biscuits. Much of Sienna's socializing occurs at night at home with her mother and the house boarders sitting in front of the television, where they chat, and enjoy the pleasures of sharing sweet foods. In the household snacking is often restrained during the day but, as Sienna explained 'after dinner it's like fair game. Everyone is just like *SNACK*!'

> If we're, you know, if we're sitting in the lounge and we're like, 'I feel like a snack,' then we get up. And then like an hour later someone else would be like, 'I feel like a snack,' and then someone will bring back other things. It's a bad system, I must admit. But that's what we do, so.

Subversive Eating

In Candy and Sienna's lounge room the experience of sweetness operates to strengthen social relations through the sharing of taste, and also by making time and space for its consumption (McLennan et al. 2014). Sweet foods, like cigarettes before them, demarcates liminal zones where everyday concerns are temporarily suspended (in tea breaks, smokos[3] and snack times) and commodities are fetishized and enjoyed. In her study on gender and class as dimensions of smoking behaviour in Britain, Graham (1994) found that cigarette smoking was associated with women from low socio-economic classes who have caring responsibilities and limited financial resources. In her study, smoking punctuated the passing of time. It was a way of marking time and making time in an otherwise chaotic or boring day. Making time in the day for oneself is promoted in the long-running Nestlé slogan that consumers should 'Have a break … have a Kit Kat', enacting self-care through momentary pleasures. In a similar light, the Australian confectionary brand Allen's reminds us that pleasure and joy, despite difficult circumstances, can be experienced in the present hence the marketing line 'It's moments like these you need Minties'.[4]

Like smoko breaks, snack-time is processual, reproducing social relations night-by-night. This intimate and relational practice of snacking in front of the television can offer an escape from the stressors of life, where the commensality of being with others either in flesh or virtually on screen is sweetened through those foods and drinks that are promoted and advertised as associated with 'enjoyment and immediate gratification' (Harris et al. 2009). Sugary products may pose 'risks' to health but they are advertised and promoted as a reward, a 'happy, sometimes secretive or 'naughty' indulgence' (McLennan et al. 2014). Candy buys large packets containing 'fun sized chocolates' or single servings of sweet biscuits such as Tiny Teddies. Asserting that 'it's more expensive that way' she pays heed to health advice by purchasing sugary foods 'in small amounts', and in line with her daughter's desire to lose weight. 'You know' Candy said 'a moment on the lips, a lifetime on the hips'. Competing paradigms of care collide as health discourses of 'careful eating' and relational practices of sweetening shape and constrain food portions and preferences. However, restraint is difficult to exercise at night when 'subversive' eating (Albon 2005) takes hold. As Sienna conveyed guiltily: 'It's a bad system, I must admit. But that's what we do'. Contested enactments of care are played out in Candy's relationship with her obese stepdad. While her own mother worries about his weight and its impact on his health, Candy sneaks him lollipops asserting 'you can't deny the man everything'.

'Subversive' eating is not only a central impetus in children's taste for sugar (Albon 2005) but is sustained into adulthood, with a sense of 'naughtiness' around the consumption of sweet foods that is promoted in the marketing of

---

3 A slang term used in Australia for a short cigarette break.
4 Minties are a soft chewable mint flavoured sweet.

ready-made sugary products (McLennan et al. 2014). In contrast, the social marketing that informs health and welfare programmes in Playford demonstrates a moral imperative to encourage people in the community to make the 'right' food decisions and, in turn, to care for themselves and their families. Care operates through food, explicitly healthy food, in obesity interventions like OPAL, but this understanding of care is contested in Candy's family where caring through food involves more than simply choosing or providing healthy options (Fox and Smith 2011).

Our ethnography reveals 'care' to be a more fluid category, and one that operates through the nuanced day-to-day sweetening of social life. Care is thus embodied and negotiated in sharing the pleasures of sugar, and, conversely, in the public health imaginings that promote its restriction. In their discourse analysis of maternal resistance to Jamie Oliver's school dinners in the working class area of Rotherham in the UK, Fox and Smith (2011) point to the ways in which media sources and government policies overlook the multiple meanings of care that are constructed and embodied in the provision of food. Shunning homemade school meals and resisting health interventions, Rotherham mothers caught media attention by passing burgers and buns to their children through the school railings. Labelled in the popular press as 'sinner ladies', the mothers came to represent the 'flawed consumption' habits and practices of the UK working classes (Peacock et al. 2014. See also Warin 2011). Resonant with tensions between the discursive framings of care in healthy lifestyle programs and the embodied practice of sweetening, the Rotherham mothers' offering of pleasant tasting foods to their children was represented in the media as a marker of 'distorted priorities' (Peacock et al. 2014). These examples point to the coalescence of class and gender in care contexts. Care through feeding is entrenched in cultural understandings of women's roles and is positioned in the media as susceptible to working-class mothers' poor 'tastes', their unhealthy diet and lifestyle choices (Fox and Smith 2011; Gillies 2007). Public health notions of careful eating compete therefore with differing paradigms of care (including powerful connections of kinship, gender relations and care through food) in places of disadvantage.

Conclusion

In the lives of our participants refined sugars are immediately satiating, easy to access and affordable. Yet they are positioned as 'sometimes' or 'discretionary foods' in government advice. Sociological literature has shown how, in the context of social disadvantage, public health care that asks people to refrain from the things that they take pleasure in 'may do more harm than good' (Lindsay 2010. See also Stead et al. 2011). The arguments in this chapter go beyond the troubling of public health configurations of 'care' that persist in nutritional discourse to demonstrate how people care through sweetening. We agree with Mol et al. that 'writing about care' requires a 'need to juggle with our language and adapt it' to everyday situations where care 'may involve jointly drinking a hot chocolate while chatting about nothing in particular' (2010b: 10). In places of poverty and hardship, we argue, 'tinkering' with food, eating and bodies is instrumental to the sweetening of circumstances and social relations.

Our research on sweetening has parallels with studies on the relationship between bodies, place and smoking which demonstrate a class and gendered gradient to smoking behaviour. Research conducted in a low income area in Glasgow, Scotland reveals how smoking is practised in order to deal with living in a stigmatized region (Stead et al. 2001). Similarly, studies in the UK show how socio-economic inequality contributes to the smoking activity of mothers from minority groups and in poor communities, as smoking can be associated with 'resting and refuelling'; the maintenance of usual routines; a way to cope with boredom and breakdowns in normal everyday life; a 'break' from the ongoing, intensive care of children (Graham et al. 2006; Hawkins et al. 2010; Marsh and McKay 1994). In research conducted in Christchurch, New Zealand the double stigma of living in a socially disadvantaged neighbourhood and the habit of smoking (a stigmatizing activity) creates 'smoking islands' in which smoking is a normalized behaviour (Thompson et al. 2007). Similarly, our fieldwork demonstrates that sweetening operates among research participants living in Playford both as a visceral technique and as an everyday form of resistance, for ameliorating 'inequalities in the social trajectories in which they are embedded' (Graham et al. 2006: 7).

Healthy lifestyle programs in Playford face challenges when the eating habits of people are unresponsive to health messages, which can be undermined by making them amenable to people's own agendas or identities. This 'normative dissonance' (Popay et al. 2013) is played out in the living room of Candy who consumes 'fun size' chocolates because they are 'in small amounts'. It is also embodied in the lives of Sienna and Jude who deploy sweetening as a strategy for experiencing, albeit momentarily, the comfort and happiness that are eroded in personal histories of rejection, abuse, bullying, depression, and anxiety. Assigning a positive value to sugar and sweetness is a technique used by this marginalized group to 'upset sensory and social hierarchies' (Howes and Classen 2014: 77) entrenched in mainstream public health campaigns that construct sugar as wholly negative. We propose that sweetening must be understood in its local context, as embedded in the bodies and social lives of those who sweeten in order to cope and to care when one's place in the world diminishes possibilities for other securities (Peacock et al. 2014). Public health imperatives to reduce sugar consumption (and its multiple meanings) among those with what Graham et al. term 'biographies of disadvantage' (2006: 7) may be marred then by the efforts and practices of the disenfranchized to make social life palatable, in effect, to make the bitter sweet.

Acknowledgements

This project was funded by an Australian Research Council Grant (LP 120100155). South Australia Health (Government of South Australia) and the City of Playford have contributed funds and in-kind support for this project. We wish to thank our participants for the time they took to share their views and experiences with us.

Disclaimer: The views expressed in this publication do not necessarily reflect South Australian Government Policies.

References

Ahmed, U. 2013. Bro, are you selling? *Curiosity Creative* [online]. Available at: http://vimeo.com/63830797 [accessed: 17 July 2014].

Albon, D.J. 2005. Approaches to the study of children, food and sweet eating: A review of the literature. *Early Child Development and Care*, 175(5), 407-17.

Barnes, M. 2010. *Care in Everyday Life: An Ethic of Care in Practice*. Bristol: Policy Press.

Bourdieu, P. 1977. *Outline of a Theory of Practice*. Stanford, CA: Stanford University Press.

Bourdieu, P. 1984. *Distinction: A Social Critique of the Judgement of Taste*. New York: Routledge.

Bryant, E.J., King, N.A. and Blundell, J.E. 2007. Disinhibition: Its effects on appetite and weight regulation. *Obesity Reviews*, 9(5), 409-19.

Commission on Social Determinants of Health. 2008. *CSDH Final Report: Closing the Gap in a Generation: Health Equity through Action on the Social Determinants of Health*. Geneva: World Health Organization.

Coveney, J. 1999. The science and spirituality of nutrition. *Critical Public Health*, 9(1), 23-37.

Cowan, J. 1990. *Dance and the Body Politic in Northern Greece*. Princeton, NJ: Princeton University Press.

Cowan, J. 1991. Going out for coffee? Contesting the grounds of gendered pleasures in everyday sociability, in *Contested Identities: Gender and Kinship in Modern Greece*, edited by P. Loizos and E. Papataksiarchis. Princeton, NJ: Princeton University Press, 180-202.

de Certeau, M. 1984. *The Practice of Everyday Life*. Berkeley, CA: University of California Press.

Drewnowski, A. 2012. The economics of food choice behavior: Why poverty and obesity are linked, in *Obesity Treatment and Prevention: New Directions*, edited by A. Drewnowski and B.J. Rolls. Nestlé Nutritional Workshop Series, 73, 95-112. Available at: https://www.nestlenutrition-institute.org [accessed: 1 October 2014].

Fox, R. and Smith, G. 2011. Sinner ladies and the gospel of good taste: Geographies of food, class and care. *Health and Place*, 17(2), 403-12.

Gillies, V. 2007. *Marginalised Mothers: Exploring Working Class Experiences of Parenting*. Abingdon: Routledge.

Graham, H. 1994. Gender and class as dimensions of smoking behaviour in Britain: Insights from a survey of mothers. *Social Science and Medicine*, 38(5), 691-98.

Graham, H., Inskip, H.M., Francis, B. and Harman, J. 2006. Pathways of disadvantage and smoking careers: Evidence and policy implications. *Journal of Epidemiology and Community Health*, 60(2), 7-12.

Hall, B. 1979. Uniformity of Human Milk. *American Journal of Clinical Nutrition*, 32(2), 304-12.

Harris, J.L., Pomeranz, J.L., Lobstein, T. and Brownell, K.D. 2009. A crisis in the marketplace: how food marketing contributes to childhood obesity and what can be done. *Annual Review of Public Health*, 30(1), 211-25.

Hartwick, C.A., Coveney, J., Cox, D., Meyer, S. and Sue, R. 2014. Transferring an innovation in food and lifestyle education: Adaptation of a French obesity prevention methodology in Australia (262.2). *The Federation of American Societies for Experimental Biology Journal*, 28(1), 262-2.

Hawkins, S.S., Law, C. and Graham, H. 2010. Lifecourse influences on maternal smoking before pregnancy and postpartum among women from ethnic minority groups. *The European Journal of Public Health*, 20(3), 339-45.

Held, V. 2006. *The Ethics of Care: Personal, Political, and Global*. Oxford: Oxford University Press.

Hollingworth, S. and Williams, K. 2009. Constructions of the working-class 'Other' among urban, white, middle-class youth: 'Chavs', subculture and the valuing of education. *Journal of Youth Studies*, 12(5), 467-82.

Hordacre, A.L., Spoehr, J., Crossman, S. and Barbaro, B. 2013. *City of Playford Socio-demographic, Employment and Education Profile*. Adelaide: Australian Workplace Innovation and Social Research Centre.

Howes, D. and Classen, C. 2014. *Ways of Sensing: Understanding the Senses in Society*. London: Routledge.

Landecker, H. 2011. Food as exposure: Nutritional epigenetics and the new metabolism. *BioSocieties*, 6(2), 167-94.

Lindsay, J. 2010. Healthy living guidelines and the disconnect with everyday life. *Critical Public Health*, 20(4), 475-87.

Lock, M. 1993. Encounters with Aging: Mythologies of Menopause in Japan and North America. Berkeley, CA: University of California Press.

Lock, M. 2013. The epigenome and nature/nurture reunification: A challenge for anthropology. *Medical Anthropology*, 32(4), 291-308.

Marsh, A. and McKay, S. 1994. *Poor Smokers*. London: Institute of Policy Studies.

McLachlan, R,. Gilfillan, G. and Gordon, J. 2013. *Deep and Persistent Disadvantage in Australia*. Productivity Commission Report. Canberra: Commonwealth of Australia.

McLennan A.K., Ulijaszek S.J. and Eli, K. 2014. Social aspects of dietary sugars, in *Dietary Sugars and Health: From Biology to Policy*, edited by M.I. Goran, L. Tappy and K-A. Lê. Abingdon: Taylor and Francis.

Mennella, J.A. and Ventura, A.K. 2010. Understanding the basic biology underlying the flavor world of children. *Current Zoology*, 56(6), 834-41.

Mintz, S.W. 1985. *Sweetness and Power: The Place of Sugar in Modern History*. New York: Penguin Books.

Mol, A. 2008. *The Logic of Care: Health and the Problem of Patient Choice*. London: Routledge.

Mol, A. 2010. Care and its values: Good food in the nursing home, in *Care in Practice: On Tinkering in Clinics, Homes and Farms*, edited by A. Mol et al. New London: Transaction Publishers, 215-34.

Mol, A., Moser, I. and Pols, J. 2010a. *Care in Practice: On Tinkering in Clinics, Homes and Farms*. New London: Transaction Publishers.

Mol, A, Moser, I. and Pols, J. 2010b. Care: Putting practice into theory, in *Care in Practice: On Tinkering in Clinics, Homes and Farms*, edited by A. Mol, I. Moser and J. Pols. New London: Transaction Publishers, 7-26.

National Health and Medical Research Council. 2013. *Eat For Health: Australian Dietary Guidelines*. 1 October 2014 [Online]. Available at: http://www.eatforhealth.gov.au/sites/default/files/files/the_guidelines/n55_australian_dietary_guidelines.pdf [accessed: 1 October 2014].

Nayak, A. 2006. Displaced masculinities: Chavs, youth and class in the post-industrial city. *Sociology*, 40(5), 813-31.

Niewöhner, J. 2011. Epigenetics: Embedded bodies and the molecularisation of biography and milieu. *BioSocieties*, 6(3), 279-98.

Offer, A., Pechey, R. and Ulijaszek, S. 2012. *Insecurity, Inequality, and Obesity in Affluent Societies*. Oxford: Oxford University Press.

Peacock, M., Bissell, P. and Owen, J. 2014. Shaming encounters: Reflections on contemporary understandings of social inequality and health. *Sociology*, 48(2), 387-402.

Pearce, J., Barnett, R. and Moon, G. 2012. Socio-spatial inequalities in health-related behaviours: Pathways linking place and smoking. *Progress in Human Geography*, 36(1), 3-21.

Peel, M. 2004. Imperfect bodies of the poor. *Griffith Review*, 21, 83-93.

Popay, J., Thomas, C., Williams, G., Bennett, S., Gatrell, A. and Bostock, L. 2003. A proper place to live: health inequalities, agency and the normative dimensions of space. *Social Science and Medicine*, 57(1), 55-69.

Putland, C., Baum, F.E. and Ziersch, A.M. 2011. From causes to solutions – insights from lay knowledge about health inequalities. *BMC Public Health*, 11, 1-11.

Scott, J.C. 1985. *Weapons of the Weak: Everyday Forms of Peasant Resistance*. New Haven, CT: Yale University Press.

Serematakis, C. 1994. *The Senses Still: Perception and Memory as Material Culture in Modernity*. Boulder, CO: Westview Press.

Stead, M., MacAskill, S., MacKintosh, A.M., Reece, J. and Eadie, D. 2001. 'It's as if you're locked in': Qualitative explanations for area effects on smoking in disadvantaged communities. *Health and Place*, 7(4), 333-43.

Stead, M., McDermott, L., MacKintosh, A.M. and Adamson, A. 2011. Why healthy eating is bad for young people's health: Identity, belonging and food. *Social Science and Medicine*, 72(7), 1131-39.

Stoller, P. 1989. *The Taste of Ethnographic Things*. Philadelphia, PA: University of Pennsylvania Press.

The University of Adelaide: Population Research and Outcomes Studies (PROS). 2014. Health of South Australian Adults – City of Playford. Technical Report January 2011-December 2013. Commissioned by South Australian Department for Health and Ageing; October 2014.

Thompson, L., Pearce, J. and Barnett, J.R. 2007. Moralising geographies: Stigma, smoking islands and responsible subjects. *Area*, 39(4), 508-17.

Tronto, J. 1993. *Moral Boundaries: A Political Argument for an Ethic of Care*. London: Routledge.

Ward, P.R., Verity, F., Carter, P., Tsourtos, G., Coveney, J. and Wong, K.C. 2013. Food stress in Adelaide: The relationship between low income and the affordability of healthy food. *Journal of Environmental and Public Health* 968078, 1-10 [online]. Available at: http://www.hindawi.com/journals/jeph [accessed: 1 October 2014].

Warin, M. 2011. Foucault's progeny: Jamie Oliver and the art of governing obesity. *Social Theory and Health*, 9(1), 24-40.

Warin, M and Dennis, S. 2005. Threads of memory: Reproducing the cypress tree through sensual consumption. *Journal of Intercultural Studies*, 26(1-2), 159-70.

Wilkinson, R.G. and Pickett, K. 2009. *The Spirit Level: Why More Equal Societies Almost Always Do Better*. London: Penguin.

Wong, K.C., Coveney, J., Ward, P., Muller, R., Carter, P., Verity, F. and Tsourtos, G. 2011. Availability, affordability and quality of a healthy food basket in Adelaide, South Australia. *Nutrition and Dietetics*, 68(1), 8-14.

Chapter 6

Food, Weight and Care in the Consultation

Antje Lindenmeyer

Invisibilities of Food

Interactions around food, weight and eating that take place during health care consultations can bring up complex emotions. Exploring the context for these emotions necessitates looking at, and linking, discourses and debates around food and eating, and care. Above all, Fisher and Tronto's (1990) four dimensions of care can shed light on different aspects of the consultation: On the side of the health professional, 'caring about' (attentiveness) aims to be mindful of the other's need; within the biomedical paradigm, this could be seen as the doctor or nurse noticing that the patient is overweight and therefore in need of help. However, it might be more fruitful to interpret 'caring about' as attending to the patient more holistically, without prioritizing weight. 'Caring for' implies the doctor or nurse taking on responsibility for the patient, and initiating the actual work of 'caring': the dialogue of the consultation which should include talking about food and eating in a sensitive manner. However, the care receiver is also involved by being receptive and judging the effectiveness of care. As food and eating are an important aspect of maintaining health in everyday life, 'caring about' what other people eat becomes an important aspect of 'caring for' the patient.

Setting aside the debate over whether weight loss itself is desirable, achievable in the long term or salutogenic (Aphramor 2005), this chapter initially set out to explore the entanglement of food and care in primary care consultations. I aimed to identify accounts of these consultations in the qualitative health literature to find out how doctors, nurses and patients experienced them and how 'care' was understood in this context. For this, I aimed at a broad reading rather than a systematic approach[1], with a review of qualitative and sociological journals backed up by a Medline and CINAHL search (using search terms such as weight/obesity in combination with primary care/consultation/doctor-patient relations), followed by snowballing from citations. I extracted quotes that illustrated interactions between health professionals and patients that took place during the consultations, focusing especially on emotions experienced by both parties. As many studies were quite descriptive, it was not possible to conduct a full meta-ethnography

---

1   Similar to qualitative reviews with a more systematic approach (cf. Malterud and Ulriksen 2011; Mold and Forbes 2011), most articles discussed here are from the UK, US, Australia or Scandinavian countries and the majority of participants are female and white.

drawing together authors' interpretations of what had occurred (see Thorne et al. 2004). Instead, I conducted a secondary analysis of data from participant quotes and descriptive passages, including theoretical interpretations where they were given (cf. Gronning 2013; Tischner 2013). This enabled me to draw on a wide range of sources and develop a focus on care and emotion that would have not otherwise been possible.

When working through the literature, it soon became apparent that food is a curious absence in this literature, with weight taking centre stage. Researchers looking at experiences of giving and receiving healthy eating advice have noted a curious slippage between 'healthy eating' and 'weight management', with healthy eating campaigns, dieticians, GPs and patients focusing on weight rather than what is eaten (McClinchy et al. 2013). While qualitative research has explored the complex individual meanings attached to food and eating practices, e.g. as an expression of personal memory and nostalgia (see for example Ferzacca 2004; Lupton 1994), interactions in the clinic sometimes boil down to exhortations to 'eat less':

> He said, 'Well, you just have to stop eating'. And I said, 'If it would have been easy for me, I would have done it a long time ago'. (Merrill and Grassley 2008: 143)

> I went to see my doctor and he gave me the following comment: 'Eat less and exercise more and stop complaining!' (Gronning et al. 2013: 277)

Where food does appear, it emerges as a topic that doctors and nurses use to talk about their patients. This tends to come with a strong moral framework that differentiates between good and bad foods (see Lupton 1996). For example, cream cakes and biscuits are mentioned by professionals to illustrate patients' refusal to take on board their recommendations. Meanwhile, 'good foods' are introduced to give an exaggerated picture of patients being untruthful or in denial about their eating, with patients saying they are eating nothing but fruit and vegetables or lettuce. Both these usages are unlikely to lead to a meaningful discussion about food and eating in the consultation.

To begin with, I will trace how this slippage from food to weight is encouraged by a wider stigmatizing cultural and clinical focus on a need to 'tackle' what is widely, but possibly unhelpfully, termed an 'obesity epidemic' (Flegal 2006; Mitchell and McTigue 2007). This concept frames policies and practices of care, with 'caring about' obesity shaping ways of 'caring for' patients. I will argue that caring about obesity without also caring about the complexities of food and eating creates a disconnect between what both carers and cared-for 'ought' to do and their lived realities (see also Zivkovik et al. this volume). In turn, this gives rise to difficult emotions of anger and frustration that complicate discussions around food and eating. This chapter, then, will look at the intersections between weight discussions, emotions and bodies, exploring why these discussions are so extremely uncomfortable for doctors, nurses and patients.

The 'Obesity Crisis': From Caring About to Caring For

Consultations on food and weight take place in the familiar context of obesity as a major public health crisis, with both the academic and professional literature, as well as the mass media, full of alarm on the impact of the 'obesity epidemic' (Campos 2004) and the cost especially to publicly-funded health services (Wang et al. 2011). A policy paper by the Academy of Medical Royal Colleges (2013) is one of many voices comparing the work of anti-obesity campaigners to those that championed tobacco control in earlier decades:

> Like those doctors who realised that smoke-filled homes and offices of the 1950s were creating a health time-bomb, we demand action today. Just as the challenge of persuading society that the deeply embedded habit of smoking was against its better interests, changing how we eat and exercise is now a matter of necessity.
> (Academy of Medical Royal Colleges 2013: 14)

Food choice, however, is more than just a 'deeply embedded habit'. Sociologists and anthropologists have widely explored the myriad social, ritual and interactional functions of food (see for example Lupton 1996; Visser 1986; Wilk 2010). Furthermore, while tobacco can be simply, however painfully, 'cut out', food sustains life: 'People do not need to smoke, but they do need to eat'; this common-sense statement has been used by the WHO Director-General to urge the worldwide development of healthier food environments (Chan 2011). Yet, current health policy initiatives tend to focus on the individual rather than the environment. A case in point is the UK based 'Making Every Contact Count' (MECC) which recommends that primary care professionals raise weight and eating with their overweight patients as often as possible. This means that 'caring about' what people eat could become an important part of doctors' and nurses' professional roles of 'caring for' patients.

However, a problem arises in the transition from 'caring about' to 'caring for' (officially taking on responsibility for the patient), especially when the details of that care are pre-figured by guidelines. For example, the MECC programme stresses the importance of empowering individuals and helping them to make their own decisions (see for example the training materials published by NHS Yorkshire and the Humber in 2010). Yet, it can be assumed from the overall climate of urgency that weight will often be raised regardless of the original reason for the consultation and the patient's wishes. This matters as 'caring about' includes focusing – for the moment – exclusively on intuiting what the individual person feels and needs: attentiveness (Fisher and Tronto 1990), or empathy (Mercer and Reynolds 2002). In their extensive analysis of 'kindness' in modern health care, Ballatt and Campling describe a virtuous cycle in which an underlying tenor of kindness (warmth, sympathy, compassion) can lead to attentiveness to the individual patient (noticing, thinking, feeling, learning), which in turn enables attunement (responsiveness, sensitive caring) and fosters trust and improved co-operation between patient and health professional (Ballatt and Campling 2011: 45).

Qualitative research with overweight people, however, has found that this focus on what the patient feels and needs is often not realized in practice (Chugh et al. 2013; Tischner 2013). Since raising the topics of weight and eating is framed as potentially lifesaving by health policy, accepting responsibility for the patient ('caring for') can imply that the doctor or nurse now feels responsible for the patient's eating; this leads the health professional to 'care about' obesity rather than the individual patient. This can result in 'apparently appropriate advice [being] perceived as patronising by patients' (Malterud and Ulriksen 2011).

Two exploratory frameworks are particularly valuable to contextualize the qualitative literature around consultations on weight. One very clearly is the existence of weight stigma and the 'spoiled identity' (Goffman 1963) of obesity, which will be discussed in more detail later in this chapter. The other is the embodied experience of being overweight, which is closely linked to emotions and relationships around food (Tischner 2013). Qualitative studies offer rich descriptions of emotions unleashed during consultations which, with the unequal distribution of power in the consultation (Foucault 2003; Turner 1987), could inhibit the free, empowering dialogue envisioned by MECC campaigners. The accounts of study participants also suggest that emotions are often not expressed in the consultation, especially when they are 'difficult' emotions such as anger. It is however possible to imagine that they contribute to overweight people delaying to seek help for other health problems (Mold and Forbes 2011).

The literature on doctors' and nurses' thoughts and experiences around raising weight in the consultation shows that, while many see making patients aware of their weight and the associated health risks as part of their duty to provide care (Hansson et al. 2011), some are also aware of the potential sensitivity of the topic. This could mean refraining from possibly-upsetting terms, and sometimes avoiding the topic altogether (Brown and Thompson 2007). Doctors and nurses may deliberately choose not to raise the topic of weight in order to avoid opening a 'Pandora's box of psychological problems' (Michie 2007). On the other hand, these consultations emerge as difficult spaces for all involved. Patients might feel patronized when being told what (not) to eat. However, doctors and nurses can feel vulnerable too, despite the power imbalance in the clinic discussed by Foucault and others. Trying to instigate behaviour change is often tinged with frustration when the patient does not lose weight. As weight is always visible and cannot be disguised, practitioners' own struggles with their body can come uncomfortably to the fore when discussing weight and eating.

Primary care is different from other health encounters, such as with dieticians, in that there is the potential for an ongoing discussion around weight with the same doctor or nurse. Both patients and health professionals bring the memory of earlier discussions about weight with them, and these are embedded in personal experiences over the whole lifecourse. Not only do patients often have a history of struggling with weight that goes back to their childhood, but also a history of consultations about weight (in my own case, this goes back to my mother being given a booklet titled *Your Overweight Child* when I was 13). Some patients may expect the history of past consultations to be taken into account when eating and weight is mentioned; doing so might make these discussions more fruitful and less painful.

Anger

In accounts from overweight research participants, anger towards a doctor or nurse is often palpable, emerging in the literature as well-honed stories outlining the impact of an insensitive or thoughtless remark in the consultation. As if in an attempt to diffuse the rawness of the pain felt by the teller, humour is often used when these stories are recounted. While open discrimination and humiliation by doctors or nurses is rarely recounted, weight stigma can still overshadow interactions with health professionals when the patient feels angry at being positioned as lazy and stupid:

> [Female participant]: My [overweight] friends and myself are all people who've got degrees … we can read the literature … and we fully understand what we should or shouldn't eat. (Tischner 2013: 81)

Ostensibly neutral clinical terms such as 'obese' can also provoke negative emotions (Gray et al. 2011):

> [Female participant]: 'Morbidly obese' I hate it. I hate that term. It just plays hell with my mind. I'm not morbid, I'm not ugly, I'm not a morbid person; I'm a happy person. (Thomas et al. 2008: 324)

This account shows how being labelled 'morbidly obese' can be perceived as a hurtful and anger-inducing judgement of the whole person. As hinted above, considerable annoyance may also be caused by a doctor or nurse introducing obesity without asking about the patient's history or any previous attempts to lose weight. This does not only move the consultation away from the immediate needs of the patient but also creates a disjoint between the consultation and the experience of a lifetime of struggling with weight:

> [Female participant]: The doctor said, 'Well, your blood pressure is high. You need to lose weight'. And I said, 'I realize that'. He said, 'Well, you just have to stop eating'. And I said, 'If it would have been easy for me, I would have done it a long time ago'. And he said, 'Well, you just need to learn how to do that'. And

so to me it was like an impasse … I walked out of there … and I thought, 'The hell I will!' (laugh). (Merrill and Grassley 2008: 143)

While this discussion creates a strong response of anger and rebellion, other patients recount feeling frustrated and angry by only being given standardized information without regard to past attempts at losing weight:

[Female participant]: I think if they listened and respected you as an individual instead of lumping fat women together … You should be more interested in hearing me say, 'I've tried A, B, C, and D. How do we get to G, F, H, I, J?'. (Chugh et al. 2013: 424)

[Male participant]: I went to see my doctor and he gave me the following comment: 'Eat less and exercise more and stop complaining!' I thought 'you don't understand jack shit'. I asked him if he expected me to pay for the consultation and he said yes. I told him to forget about it and I haven't seen him since. (Gronning et al. 2013: 277)

Interactions that imply a perception that every health condition is put down to a person's weight may cause not just anger, but also worry that other problems might be overlooked:

[Participant, gender unclear]: you think, 'Well, nobody's going to tell you what's wrong if you've got something wrong with you because they're putting everything down to your weight,' and to me that's wrong. (Brown et al. 2006: 670)

[Female participant]: I've had medical professionals tell me that problems I've had are because of my weight when I've had the same problems for a number of years before I was at this weight … people try and make it easy for medical professionals not to address people's actual real health problems and just say well if you go away and lose weight, you know, then you'll be better. (Tischner 2013: 91)

Both male and female participants cited above show a strong sense of anger; because anger is a difficult emotion for people in a situation of unequal power, and especially for women (Kring 2000), this may be more problematic for female patients. In the accounts above, anger is not expressed in the consultation, although some doctors and nurses recount how patients may become 'furious' if their weight is raised when they come in with an unrelated issue (Hansson et al. 2011). Nurses also realize that some patients may stay away once it becomes clear that they will be weighed (McClinchy et al. 2013).

It seems a common-sense proposition that some health professionals should respond emotionally to these consultations as well. The following accounts show health professionals feeling frustrated and annoyed as the patient does not lose weight:

> [Health professional]: But it's when you get 6 weeks down the line and they're still not losing weight and they swear blind they're eating nothing that you start the struggling and you think, well, where do we go now? (McClinchy et al. 2013: 502)

> [Male GP]: You can lead a horse to water but you can't stop it eating cream cakes. (Gunther et al. 2012: 98)

> [GP]: I end up feeling it isn't possible for them to do it [lose weight], so I feel annoyed with them for not just doing it. (Epstein and Ogden 2005: 752)

While these responses could be seen as not very 'caring', Ballatt and Campling (2011) clearly link this kind of negative feelings to discourses around care. They describe how feelings of being a failure due to an inability to make a lasting difference – compounded by a target driven work culture – can lead to dislike and resentment towards patients. As these emotions contradict the self-image of 'caring' professions, they are often not voiced and doctors and nurses can feel guilty about having them. In this context, it is 'all too easy to feel furious with patients who appear to be undermining all efforts to help them' (ibid.: 60).

  In the accounts discussed here, professionals do not openly speak of showing their anger and frustration towards patients. However, one GP does discuss using anger as a motivator:

> [Female GP]: I express frustrations to my patients sometimes. ... I think they have to see us getting a little bit upset or angry ... I think some patients are moved by that, and I think it does get them going a little bit. (Gudzune et al. 2012: 154)

Other health professionals described how they could retreat behind blocking communication and standard advice without expressing anger (ibid.), while patients might still perceive criticism from the tone of the doctor's voice:

> [Female participant]: So, you're on the receiving end of factual comments that are – the intonation is disapproving. ... It's not what you say; it's how you say it. (Chugh et al. 2013: 424)

The experiences described above are highly personal but can still be divided into two broad typologies that seem especially prone to producing anger and frustration. On the one hand, a disconnect appears between the patient's and the health professional's understanding of what is important for the consultation, for example when weight is raised out of the blue, or when other health issues are ignored in favour of weight. This means that 'caring about' obesity trumps 'caring about' the patient. On the other hand, the persistence of weight over time may wear down both health professionals and patients: 'it's an issue every time they come in' (Brown and Thompson 2007). While patients may feel that their lifelong struggle with weight is being ignored, doctors and nurses are frustrated that patients seem not to be doing enough to help themselves. However, some health professionals acknowledge that rapport and trust is built up over time, with discussions of weight a 'continuous conversation over many years' (Gudzune et al. 2012). In order to lead to the real partnership envisioned by Gudzune et al., this conversation should acknowledge a patient's lived experience of weight as well as the history of earlier discussions.

Shame, Guilt and 'Saving Face'

The stigmatized nature of obesity is acknowledged by many qualitative studies of the patient experience (see Gronning et al. 2013, Malterud and Ulriksen 2011). What makes the experience of weight stigma particularly distressing is the constant visibility of obesity. While someone who is smoking or regularly drinking alcohol may be able to 'pass' as healthy at times, the overweight body is always on display with some overweight people feeling constantly monitored, for example when eating in public or shopping for food (Tischner 2013). This phenomenon may be reinforced by the ubiquity of de-humanized representations of 'headless fatties' in the media (Cooper 2007). The moral implications of obesity, its conflation with gluttony and laziness and its use as a vehicle for uneasiness with a society driven by growth and consumption (see for example Bordo 2003), work to position the overweight person as morally deficient. This can take the form of the body as 'metonymically' standing for the whole person which is then seen as morally deficient (Tischner 2013: 115). Overweight people interviewed about their experiences often stress that they are more than 'just' their weight but that they feel judged by other members of the public: 'People think you're stupid. If you're fat you're stupid or you're a pig ... you're a glutton. You gorge yourself' (Brown et al. 2006: 669).

When applying the concept of weight stigma to health interactions, some researchers focus on health professionals' stigmatizing attitudes which, although not always conscious or directly expressed, can lead to patients experiencing labelling, stereotyping or discrimination. This, in turn, may render patients avoiding healthcare or screening (Malterud and Ulriksen 2011; Mold and Forbes 2011). On the other hand, some doctors and nurses were seen to respond compassionately to their patients' distress:

> [Female GP]: There comes a time when you get so disappointed with yourself, because you just can't lose weight. You think you've done everything, and you still can't like yourself. You lose confidence. (Hansson et al. 2011: 8)

The concept of stigma resulting in a 'spoiled identity' (Goffman 1963) could be instrumental in understanding why some patients readily accept that only they are to blame for their weight and any medical conditions possibly related to it (Malterud and Ulriksen 2011), while others attempt to resist the stigmatized identity (Tischner 2013). Gronning and colleagues (2013) link obesity stigma to Goffman's theory of a split between a socially acceptable, visible 'front stage' and an invisible, private 'back stage' persona (Goffman 1969) to explore how overweight people manage shame and blame. As weight is always visible, it cannot be hidden back stage; however, people can avoid presenting themselves as lazy and greedy by explaining their weight problem through factors over which they have little or no control, such as physical or mental problems (Gronning et al. 2013: 274). Others may portray themselves as 'addicted' to food or not in control of their eating as their families reject foods they dislike (see for example Peel et al. 2005). However, doctors may interpret a self-presentation as powerless as pushing responsibility towards *them*:

> [GP]: I think a lot of them believe that someone else is going to do the job for them. ... They put the responsibility on me; I'm the one who's going to fix it so they lose weight. (Hansson et al. 2011: 7)

As the stigmatized identity of obesity is strongly linked to ideas of responsibility for the self, some overweight people resist stigma by positioning themselves as a 'responsible fat person' who engages in activities seen as healthy in a medical paradigm, such as keeping fit or eating lots of vegetables (Tischner 2013: 77). Taking this position can also lead to the consultation becoming difficult as health professionals believe that the patient would surely lose weight if they behaved in this way:

> [Nurse]: He tells me that he eats nothing but fruit and vegetables, and that he can't understand why he hasn't lost any weight ... when a patient says that to you, it's very difficult to say, 'Look, I don't necessarily believe what you're telling me because, if you did all that, you'd be losing weight'. (Brown and Thompson 2007: 538)

> [Nurse]: They often say 'I don't understand it, I don't eat anything', but actually we know they do. (Hansson et al. 2011: 7)

> [GP]: ... almost a classic response from women who want to lose weight, but are big, is the sort of 'but I only eat a lettuce leaf' approach. (Epstein and Ogden 2005: 752)

These accounts outline a disconnect between patients' narratives and what the professional 'sees' and 'knows'. Instead of exploring what patients mean by their statements and understanding attempts to save face and avoid shame, health professionals seem to interpret them as being untruthful. This, in turn, can lead to the consultation becoming even more difficult as they do not wish to confront the patient with accusations of lying. The hyperbole in recounting unrealistic patient narratives ('only a lettuce leaf') seems to express a great deal of frustration. The following account in which a GP recalls discussing eating with people who have recently consulted a dietician is very telling in this context:

> [GP]: [The patient said] 'Well, [the dietician] said I'm doing fine' and you can see on the screen 'cut down on cakes and biscuits'. The interpretation of what's been said to them which has been a clear message and they come to me with they are 'doing fine', they never come to me and say 'they said I should eat less fat' or 'I should stop having chocolate'. They say, 'they told me to eat regularly'. (McClinchy et al. 2013: 502)

Here, the GP seems to interpret the patient's narratives as wilfully ignoring professional advice, which is especially glaring as the message given by the dietician is clearly visible 'on the screen' (again, there is a difference between what the patient says and what the professional sees). However, they can be interpreted differently, for example as focusing on positive messages ('doing fine'; 'eat regularly') while avoiding negative messages ('cutting down' 'eating less' or 'stopping'). Following Gronning et al. (2013), it could also be seen as an attempt to save face (would anyone gladly report to their doctor that they were told to stop eating chocolate?)

The accounts cited in this section illustrate how feelings of shame and attempts to save face can make consultations around weight very fraught. A focus on visible and measurable weight serves to obscure lived complexities around eating. Health professionals privileging the visible and measurable weight and the report on the computer screen may set up an antagonistic relationship with their patients who feel that their struggles with weight or to achieve a healthier life are ignored (see Tischner 2013):

> This construction [by health professionals] of obese people as fundamentally unreliable, and even deceitful, fails to take account of the shame and guilt which might inhibit full disclosure of consumption, but also discredits people's lived experiences and beliefs of their own bodies as responding differently to food. (Throsby 2007: 1565)

Many doctors and nurses seem to find it difficult to find space for 'caring about' as the need to 'care for' patients, e.g. by preventing cardiovascular disease, looms large. Doctors' accounts tend to focus on the concept of responsibility (describing attempts at saving face as denying responsibility or even pushing responsibility on to them). An additional dynamic seems to operate between doctors and nurses, with GPs feeling that patients look to them to 'fix' their problem (Hansson et al. 2011), and nurses in turn feeling frustrated that GPs offload responsibility onto them, leaving them in the role of intermediary between doctors and patients (Mercer and Tessier 2001; Wright 1998). However, some health professionals are able to discuss the often psychological reasons for being overweight rather than focusing on responsibility:

> [Health professional]: I tend to talk quite a bit about the psychology: a lot of them know what they're doing wrong but they just can't stop doing it. (McClinchy et al. 2013: 502)

> [Female GP]: It's very much a question of comforting words or, so to speak, off-loading the blame. (Hansson et al. 2011: 6)

Doctors and nurses taking this approach might make the consultation less likely to lead to the feelings of guilt, shame and frustration described above. Meanwhile, for patients, removing the link between talking about weight and feelings of guilt and shame could make it easier to seek a frank and open discussion of eating, thereby reducing the invisibility of food.

Visible Embodiment in the Consultation Relationship

As discussed above, another important aspect of obesity is its visibility, not only in the literature, as noted, but also corporeally. In the consultation, the doctor or nurse is given an immediate cue for questions about weight (and possibly also for the assumption that the patient is not aware that they are overweight as they would aim to lose weight if they were):

> [Nurse]: Every time they come in, it's an issue, is very demoralizing for the patient and probably negative to the relationship we have with them. (Brown and Thompson 2007: 478)

However, discussions of weight also put the body of the doctor or nurse centre stage. This can work to unsettle the 'affectively neutral' doctor role highlighted by classical medical sociology which is non-emotional and non-judgmental (Bury and Monaghan 2013); this implies that the doctors is perceived as disembodied while the body of the patient is foregrounded as an object of examination and treatment.[2] A focus on the body of the health professional becomes especially difficult if they are themselves overweight as it is increasingly seen as their responsibility to be of

---

2 Some sociologists have also outlined a gendered dimension to this dynamic, in which the doctor's role is aligned with rationality and masculinity (DasGupta 2003), whereas the role of the nurse is more complex as there is a strong link to caring for the body of the patient and taking on a maternal role (Allan 2005).

a normal weight (Monaghan 2010). Therefore, the authority of the doctor or nurse as expert could suffer if they were seen not to follow their own advice:

> [Male participant]: If [the practitioner] were themselves in shape and fit and healthy and enthusiastic and driven and happy within themselves, I think that would all paint a picture of someone who is a success at what they are preaching. (Leske et al. 2012: 312)

Brown and Thompson's (2007) study of the impact of nurses' own body size on their interactions with obese patients provides additional examples of the uncomfortableness of nurses' embodied presence. Similar to the overweight patient who discerns criticism in the doctor's voice, the gaze of patients can affect the nurse's self-image and confidence without anything being said:

> [Nurse]: With some patients, talking about healthier eating issues, I can see them focus on my stomach ... I do feel very conscious of and sometimes I think maybe I should just move into something and go and do something else where I don't have to feel self-conscious. (Brown and Thompson 2007: 540)

Some overweight nurses aim to overcome this by discussing their own struggles with weight in an attempt to create rapport with patients (Brown and Thompson 2007; Gudzune et al. 2012). This could be a positive example for 'caring about' patients as sharing the struggle with weight also acknowledges lived realities and implies that it is a long-term process. However, there is also the worrying possibility that rapport-building between nurses and female patients may reinforce gendered stereotypes along similar lines to 'fat talk'. First described by Nichter (2000), 'fat talk' is self-depreciating discussion of weight which creates rapport in social interactions between women or girls. The flip-side is that self-esteem is reduced and beauty norms are uncritically perpetuated. In discussions between nurses and patients, these patterns could possibly work to endanger rapport rather than enhancing it: Brown and Thompson suggest that nurses who are critical of their own weight might be, in turn, more critical of their patients.

While a similarity between health professionals' and patients' weight could uncomfortably blur the boundaries between them as well as creating rapport, thin health professionals might be seen as not able to understand patients' struggles:

> [Nurse]: If they don't perceive you as ever having a problem with weight or with what you eat, then they obviously think you can't possibly understand what I'm, you know, on about. So it can be difficult. (Brown and Thompson 2007: 539)

The visual nature of the body then sets up the potential of caring relationships such as these developing into no-win situations in which the body of the health professional is always 'wrong': if they are overweight, their authority could suffer and their advice could be taken less seriously. If they are not overweight, they could be seen as unable to understand a patient's situation, thereby increasing the distance between them. On the other hand, creating rapport over weight issues could also be problematic as similarities between nurses and patients may be too easily assumed (Brown and Thompson 2007).

Compassion

So far, I have focused on emotions that make consultations around weight difficult, especially where the interaction produces strong responses such as anger or frustration in both patients and health professionals. Yet, the literature also shows that these situations can be at least partly overcome by doctors and nurses showing compassion for the patient. Similar to the 'kindness' described by Ballatt and Campling (2011), compassion is an underlying ethos of care closely linked to 'caring about' the patient, closely attending to their need as a fellow human being (Bradshaw 2011).[3] However, as compassion also has an emotional component, it can be difficult to sustain, especially towards people that seem unwilling or unable to improve their own health. Some argue that the obesity discourse increases its status as a 'self-inflicted' condition and therefore makes it harder to feel compassion for the overweight (Fraser et al. 2010; Magliocca et al. 2005). Clearly, its absence can be acutely felt by some overweight people:

> [Female participant]: Educate the doctors how we feel. Do a video letting them look, this is the way that we feel. I'm a full-figured woman, but I have feelings. I care. I want you to care. (Chugh et al. 2013: 424)

However, the difficulty of compassion might also be linked to the particular dynamics of the doctor-patient relationship in primary care, not least when there is no opportunity to resolve the problem:

> Once the person says, 'well, I'd like some help to lose weight but actually I don't want [referral to commercial weight loss programmes]' then you're absolutely right the cupboard is bare. (Aveyard 2014: no page)

Chew-Graham and colleagues (2004) argue that patients who seem unable or unwilling to summon the motivation to recover are particularly toxic for the doctor-

---

3   As compassion has been included into official health policy for nurses (Commissioning Board Chief Nursing Officer 2012), there now is the thorny question of whether it can be trained and tested; it might even constitute emotional labour if prescribed by official bodies (see for example Aldridge 1994). Ann Bradshaw (2009) describes it as a virtue, i.e. a synergy of intention and practice aimed towards care for the stranger; this is a definition I would like to use here as it is closely linked to Fisher and Tronto's (1990) description of care as both personal 'caring-about' and practical/institutional 'caring-for'.

patient relationship, as they make GPs feel powerless to bring about positive change. Moreover, an unrealistic emphasis on a good personal relationship between doctors and patients only adds to the pain and frustration for GPs who are unable to achieve it. This pattern is similar to the cycle of emotional overinvestment in the caring role, followed by negative feelings towards patients and guilt about these feelings described by Ballatt and Campling (2011). However, others claim that, given the right tools, doctors and nurses can overcome this impasse by acknowledging and validating difficult emotions (both their own and those of their patients) and negotiating solutions in partnership with the patient (Cannarella Lorenzetti et al. 2013, Halpern 2007). In the context of consultations around weight, this could move the consultation towards a focus on lived experience which should include a discussion of lived realities of food and eating; however this is likely to rely on an ongoing relationship as there is very little time in the individual consultation.

A Different Conversation?

Any conclusions regarding what is happening 'in the consultation' drawn from published qualitative research obviously need to be treated with caution. As I was looking for anything related to discussions around food and emotions during consultations in articles often focusing on other issues, I needed to 'cherry pick' passages and quotes that are illuminating in this context. Most researchers look at either health professionals or patients in isolation; while some studies draw on accounts from both, they do not elicit reflections on a shared consultation. There are publications in other fields that illustrate how this could work, for example Green et al.'s (2009) in-depth exploration of one doctor's and her patient's interpretation of what was seen and said when they discussed a breast ultrasound image. Throughout the literature there are plenty of examples of good care, either framed as compassion or as a creative tinkering and problem-solving process as described by Mol (2009). However, trying to talk about food and weight can be an intensely uncomfortable situation for both health professionals and patients, often ending with the patient not feeling 'cared for'.

While I have described the development of clashing emotional responses above, these need to be set in the context of power in the consultation. Classically, 'the clinic' has been theorized as empowering the doctor who enacts power by 'his' dehumanizing gaze (Foucault 2003) or performs a role of parental authority towards a childlike patient (Parsons 1951). This could be exacerbated by patients feeling treated like naughty children and therefore regaining a sense of autonomy by disregarding health professionals' recommendations (Broom and Whittaker 2004). However, the picture here is more complex as doctors, nurses and patients are restricted by external social forces (guidelines, time allotted for the consultation) and more recent theories also focus more on interactional and relational forms of power. In Kwok-Fu Wong's (2003) four-part model of power, the traditional understanding of power flowing from the professional is related to the most 'negative' force of power (power-over). As the gatekeeper to further treatment, the GP has some power over the patient, which becomes noticeable from patients' fears that valid health concerns may be overlooked because of an overwhelming focus on weight. The situation becomes more equalized when looking at power-to (to act or effect change) as health professionals have power to advise and the patient equally has the power to ignore advice; however, this can be a very negative power that does not affect the professional very strongly and can lead to 'irritability and dysfunctional frustration for a considerable amount of time' (Tuckett 1976: 192).

The more positive forms of power (power-from-within and power-with) are more difficult to attain in this situation. Firstly, power-from-within requires the development of self-confidence and self-acceptance that is diametrically opposed to the dynamics of weight stigma; secondly, power-with requires solidarity and therefore mutual support by overweight people or a strong collaborative relationship. This is seen in some of the health professionals' and patients' accounts but does not seem the norm for discussions of food and weight. What appears more pervasive is a dynamic of enacted powerlessness on both sides, leading to stagnation and frustration, where obesity itself seems to hold the greatest power. This can only be exacerbated by the discourse of obesity as an existential crisis with health bodies and politicians urging that 'something must be done'. On the other hand, there are opportunities for starting 'a different conversation':

> [GPs] might say, 'well it would help your blood pressure if you lost weight or you'd help prevent a heart attack if you lost weight' … probably the most helpful thing you can do … is to say, 'would you like some help to lose weight?' And then you're into a kind of a different conversation. (Aveyard 2014: no page)

While this approach moves away from using negative motivation and threat to achieve lifestyle change, it still assumes that patients will want or need 'help' and that the GP can provide it. In contrast, Iona Heath, a general practitioner well known in the UK as a strong critic of over-zealous intervention, has described 'the art of doing nothing' as essential to her role:

> I met a young doctor [who] is also a brilliant musician … she had written a piece of electronica music that she played for us. It had a repeating line … 'I know I can see you through this'. As this phrase repeated in the music, I slowly realized how different this statement is from the more usual 'I know I can help you with this' and the difference is about witnessing and about being there when there is little help to be had. It is an offer of companionship, of solidarity and a promise not to run away. It is part of the art of doing nothing. (Heath 2012: 244)

The 'art of doing nothing' includes thinking, waiting, listening, noticing, 'being present' as a compassionate human being and acknowledging that sometimes the practitioner cannot 'help', for example because the sources of the problem lie in the socio-economic environment and not the individual. In the case of consultations around food and weight, a 'doing-nothing' approach might include listening to the patient's history around food and being genuinely interested in the meaning of food in their life. It may also include political campaigning for a less obesogenic environment as 'we have an obligation to speak out for those who have no voice and to describe to politicians and policy-makers, as often as we can, how their policies play out in the realities of daily life' (ibid.: 244).

Another approach to take would be to enact a paradigm shift away from a 'weight centred framework' that seems to be effective only in the short term while leading to negative consequences such as weight cycling and other health goals being ignored (Aphramor 2005). Bacon and Aphramor (2011) have argued that a 'Health at Every Size' approach should focus on improving health by helping patients to build healthy eating and physical activity into their everyday lives, regardless of weight. A similar solution has been proposed for diabetes care:

> We find that if physicians view themselves as experts whose job is to get patients to behave in ways that reflect that expertise, both will continue to be frustrated. However, when health professionals let go of the traditional view of provider-centred care and recognize the patient as the primary decision-maker, they become more effective practitioners. (Funnell and Anderson 2000: 1709)

I started this chapter with an interest in the links between discourses of food and care and the dynamics played out in the consultation. This was grounded both in my own experience and the existing qualitative research on overweight people's perspectives. I found that interactions around weight could be intensely uncomfortable as they can unleash emotional responses in both health professionals and patients and have the potential for a mutual enactment of powerlessness in the face of obesity. Discourses of care are crucial to understanding why this happens. Unrealistic demands on the 'caring' professions could lead to exhaustion and becoming unable to care. 'Caring for' the patient is often dominated by struggles around assigning responsibility for obesity (to the patient, doctor or nurse). This means that 'caring about' the patient is superseded by modes of 'caring for' the patient dominated by attempts to effect behaviour change with little regard for the emotional aspects of food and the lived experience of being overweight. A way out of this impasse could be a focus on 'caring with', an underlying ethos of solidarity and trust between carer and cared-for (Tronto 2013) . 'Caring with' includes letting go of trying to make patients lose weight and moving from an intervention centred framework to a focus on the individual history and experience (including earlier discussions about weight). This would hopefully open the way to a real conversation about food and eating in the consultation.

References

Academy of Medical Royal Colleges 2013. *Measuring Up: The Medical Profession's Prescription for the Nation's Obesity Crisis.* London: Academy of Medical Royal Colleges.

Aldridge, M. 1994. Unlimited liability? Emotional labour in nursing and social work. *Journal of Advanced Nursing,* 20(4), 722-8.

Allan, H. 2005. Gender and embodiment in nursing: The role of the female chaperone in the infertility clinic. *Nursing Inquiry,* 12(3), 175-83.

Aphramor, L. 2005. Is a weight-centred health framework salutogenic? Some thoughts on unhinging certain dietary ideologies. *Social Theory and Health,* 3(4), 315-40.

Aveyard, P. 2014. Interview with Mark Porter. *Inside Health.* Broadcast by Radio 4 on 8th April 2014; 21.00.

Bacon, L. and Aphramor, L. 2011. Weight science: Evaluating the evidence for a paradigm shift. *Nutrition Journal,* 10:9.

Ballatt, J. and Campling, P. 2011. *Intelligent Kindness: Reforming the Culture of Healthcare.* London: RCPsych Publications.

Bordo, S. 2003. *Unbearable Weight: Feminism, Western Culture, and the Body.* Berkeley/Los Angeles/London: University of California Press.

Bradshaw, A. 2009. Measuring nursing care and compassion: The McDonaldised nurse? *Journal of Medical Ethics,* 35(8), 465-8.

Bradshaw, A. 2011. Compassion: What history teaches us. *Nursing Times,* 107(19-20), 12-4.

Broom, D. and Whittaker, A. 2004. Controlling diabetes, controlling diabetics: Moral language in the management of diabetes type 2. *Social Science and Medicine,* 58(11), 2371-82.

Brown, I. and Thompson, J. 2007. Primary care nurses' attitudes, beliefs and own body size in relation to obesity management. *Journal of Advanced Nursing,* 60(5), 535-43.

Brown, I., Thompson, J., Tod, A. and Jones, G. 2006. Primary care support for tackling obesity: A qualitative study of the perceptions of obese patients. *British Journal of General Practice,* 56(530), 666-72.

Bury, M. and Monaghan, L.F. 2013. The sick role, in *Key Concepts in Medical Sociology,* edited by J. Gabe and L.F. Monaghan. Los Angeles/London: Sage, 90-4.

Campos, P. 2004. *The Obesity Myth: Why America's Obsession with Weight is Hazardous to Your Health.* New York: Gotham Books.

Cannarella Lorenzetti, R., Jacques, M., Donovan, C. Cottrell, S. and Buck, J. 2013. Managing difficult encounters: Understanding physician, patient, and situational factors. *American Family Physician,* 87(6), 419-25.

Chan, M. 2011. The rise of chronic noncommunicable diseases: An impending disaster. Opening remarks of the Director General at the WHO Global Forum:

Addressing the Challenge of Noncommunicable Diseases. Moscow, Russian Federation, 27 April 2011.

Chew-Graham, C.A., May, C.R. and Roland, M.O. 2004. The harmful consequences of elevating the doctor-patient relationship to be a primary goal of the general practice consultation. *Family Practice*, 21(3), 229-31.

Chugh, M., Friedman, A.M., Clemow, L.P. and Ferrante, J.M. 2013. Women weigh in: Obese African American and white women's perspectives on physicians' roles in weight management. *Journal of the American Board of Family Medicine*, 26(4), 421-8.

Commissioning Board Chief Nursing Officer. 2012. *Compassion in Practice – Nursing, Midwifery and Care Staff: Our Vision and Strategy.* London: Department of Health.

Cooper, C. 2007. *Headless Fatties* [Online]. Available at: http://charlottecooper.net/publishing/digital/headless-fatties-01-07 [accessed: 14 October 2014].

Dasgupta, S. 2003. Reading bodies, writing bodies: Self-reflection and cultural criticism in a narrative medicine curriculum. *Literature and Medicine*, 22(2), 241-56.

Epsteain, L. and Ogden, E. 2005. A qualitative study of GPs' views of treating obesity. *British Journal of General Practice*, 55(519), 750-4.

Ferzacca, S. 2004. Lived food and judgments of taste at a time of disease. *Medical Anthropology*, 23(1), 41-67.

Fisher, B. and Tronto, J. 1990. Toward a feminist theory of caring, in *Circles of Care. Work and Identity in Women's Lives*, edited by E. Abel and M. Nelson. Albany, NY: State University of New York Press, 35-62.

Flegal, K.M. 2006. Commentary: The epidemic of obesity – what's in a name? *International Journal of Epidemiology*, 35(1), 72-4; discussion 81-2.

Foucault, M. 2003. *The Birth of the Clinic: An Archaeology of Medical Perception.* London: Routledge.

Fraser, S., Mahera, J. and Wright, J. 2010. Between bodies and collectivities: Articulating the action of emotion in obesity epidemic discourse. *Social Theory & Health*, 8(2), 192-209.

Funnell, M. and Anderson, R. 2000. The problem with compliance in diabetes. *Journal of the American Medical Association (JAMA)*, 284(13), 1709.

Goffman, E. 1963. *Stigma: Notes on the Management of Spoiled Identity.* New Jersey: Prentice-Hall.

Goffman, E. 1969. *The Presentation of Self in Everyday Life.* Harmondsworth: Penguin.

Gray, C.M., Hunt, K., Lorimer, K., Anderson, A.S., Benzeval, M. and Wyke, S. 2011. Words matter: A qualitative investigation of which weight status terms are acceptable and motivate weight loss when used by health professionals. *BMC Public Health*, 11, 513.

Green, E., Griffiths, F. and Lindenmeyer, A. 2009. 'It can see into your body': Gender, ICTs and decision making about midlife women's health, in *Gender* on the Line? Health Information Technologies in Context, edited by E. Balka, E. Green and F. Henwood. Basingstoke: Palgrave MacMillan, 157-76.

Gronning, I., Scambler, G. and Tjora, A. 2013. From fatness to badness: The modern morality of obesity. *Health: An Interdisciplinary Journal for the Social Study of Health, Illness and Medicine*, 17(3), 266-83.

Gudzune, K.A., Clark, J.M., Appel, L.J. and Bennett, W.L. 2012. Primary care providers' communication with patients during weight counseling: A focus group study. *Patient Education and Counseling*, 89(1), 152-7.

Gunther, S., Guo, F., Sinfield, P., Rogers, S. and Baker, R. 2012. Barriers and enablers to managing obesity in general practice: A practical approach for use in implementation activities. *Quality in Primary Care*, 20(2), 93-103.

Halpern, J. 2007. Empathy and patient-physician conflicts. *Journal of General Internal Medicine*, 22(5), 696-700.

Hansson, L., Rasmussen, F. and Ahlstrom, G. 2011. General practitioners' and district nurses' conceptions of the encounter with obese patients in primary health care. *BMC Family Practice*, 12(7), 1-10.

Heath, I. 2012. The art of doing nothing. *The European Journal of General Practice*, 18(4), 242-6.

Kring, A. 2000. Gender and anger, in *Gender and Emotion*, edited by A.H. Fischer. Cambridge: Cambridge University Press, 211-31.

Leske, S., Strodl, E. and Hou, X-Y. 2012. Patient-practitioner relationships desired by overweight/obese adults. *Patient Education and Counseling*, 89(2), 309-15.

Lupton, D. 1994. Food, memory and meaning: The symbolic and social nature of food events. *The Sociological Review*, 42(4), 664-85.

Lupton, D. 1996. *Food, the Body and the Self*. London: Sage.

Magliocca, K.R., Jabero, M.F., Alto, D.L. and Magliocca, J.F. 2005. Knowledge, beliefs, and attitudes of dental and dental hygiene students toward obesity. *Journal of Dental Education*, 69(12), 1332-9.

Malterud, K. and Ulriksen, K. 2011. Obesity, stigma, and responsibility in health care: A synthesis of qualitative studies. *International Journal of Qualitative Studies on Health and Well-being*, 6(4), 1-11.

McClinchy, J., Dickinson, A., Barron, D. and Thomas, H. 2013. Practitioner and patient experiences of giving and receiving healthy eating advice. *British Journal of Community Nursing*, 18(10), 498, 500-4.

Mercer, S.W. and Reynolds, W.J. 2002. Empathy and quality of care. *British Journal of General Practice*, 52, S9-12.

Mercer, S.W. and Tessier, S. 2001. A qualitative study of general practitioners' and practice nurses' attitudes to obesity management in primary care. *Health Bulletin*, 59(4), 248-53.

Merrill, E. and Grassley, J. 2008. Women's stories of their experiences as overweight patients. *Journal of Advanced Nursing*, 64(2), 139-46.

Michie, S. 2007. Talking to primary care patients about weight: A study of GPs and practice nurses in the UK. *Psychology, Health and Medicine*, 12(5), 521-5.

Mitchell, G.R. and McTigue, K.M. 2007. The US obesity 'epidemic': Metaphor, method, or madness? *Social Epistemiology*, 21(4), 391-423.

Mol, A. 2009. Living with diabetes: Care beyond choice and control. *Lancet*, 373 (9677), 1756-7.

Mold, F. and Forbes, A. 2011. Patients' and professionals' experiences and perspectives of obesity in health-care settings: A synthesis of current research. *Health Expectations*, 16(2), 119-42.

Monaghan, L.F. 2010. 'Physician heal thyself', part 2: Debating clinicians' bodyweight. *Social Theory and Health*, 8(1), 28-50.

NHS Yorkshire and the Humber. *Prevention and Lifestyle Behaviour Change: A Competence Framework* [online]. Available at: http://www.makingeverycontactcount.co.uk [accessed: 14 October 2014].

Nichter, M. 2000. *Fat Talk: What Girls and Their Parents Say About Dieting*. Harvard: University Press.

Parsons, T. 1951. Illness and the role of the physician: A sociological perspective. *American Journal of Orthopsychiatry*, 21(3), 452-60.

Peel, E., Parry, O., Douglas, M. and Lawton, J. 2005. Taking the biscuit? A discursive approach to managing diet in type 2 diabetes. *Journal of Health Psychology*, 10(6), 779-91.

Thomas, S.L., Hyde, J., Karunaratne, A., Herbert, D. and Komesaroff, P.A. 2008. Being 'fat' in today's world: A qualitative study of the lived experiences of people with obesity in Australia. *Health Expectations*, 11(4), 321-30.

Thorne, S., Jensen, L., Kearney M.H., Noblit, G. and Sandelowski, M. 2004. Qualitative metasynthesis: Reflections on methodological orientation and ideological agenda. *Qualitative Health Research*, 14(10), 1342-65.

Throsby, K. 2007. 'How could you let yourself get like that?' Stories of the origins of obesity in accounts of weight loss surgery. *Social Science & Medicine*, 65(8), 1561-71.

Tischner, I. 2013. *Fat Lives: A Feminist Psychological Exploration.* Hove/New York: Routledge.

Tronto, J. 2013. *Caring Democracy: Markets, Equality, and Justice.* New York: New York University Press.

Tuckett, D. 1976. Doctors and patients, in *An Introduction to Medical Sociology*, edited by D. Tuckett. London: Tavistock Press, 190-224.

Turner, B.S. 1987. *Medical Power and Social Knowledge.* London: Sage.

Visser, R. 1986. *Much Depends on Dinner: The Extraordinary History and Mythology, Allure and Obsessions, Perils and Taboos, of an Ordinary Meal.* London: Penguin.

Wang, Y.C., McPherson, K., Marsh, T., Gortmaker, S.L. and Brown, M. 2011. Health and economic burden of the projected obesity trends in the USA and the UK. *Lancet*, 378(9793), 815-25.

Wilk, R. 2010. Power at the table: Food fights and Happy Meals. *Cultural Studies, Critical Methodologies*, 10(6), 428-36.

Wong, K-F. 2003. Empowerment as a panacea for poverty – old wine in new bottles? Reflections on the World Bank's conception of power. *Progress in Development Studies*, 3(4), 307-22.

Wright, J. 1998. Female nurses' perceptions of acceptable female body size: An exploratory study. *Journal of Clinical Nursing*, 7(4), 307-15.

PART III
Caring to Eat: Distances and (Dis)Connects

This final part turns its attention to how care performs and provokes eating. Reflecting on the Part I, where eating was shown to produce relations of care, the chapters in this part now reverse that focus to demonstrate not only how care is employed to frame, generate and suffuse food and eating, but also how this framing functions to establish (particular) foods as fair, right and good. Caring about food, and foods that are cared about, are further shown as placed – into agendas, ideologies and locations – so as to support regulatory systems and the personal visions of what careful food is, how it is perceived and how it should be organized. Approaching this overall theme from diverging perspectives, all three chapters work to illustrate how assertions that claim to care-about food are mobilized in association with notions of wider moral beneficence. In so doing, they demonstrate how frameworks of care enact and inform eating behaviours in multiple settings such as the market place, social institutions and on the Internet. Consequently, these chapters also highlight the ways in which careful food is simultaneously constructed as safe and fair food – meaning, in this context, food that supports and sustains all parties involved. As such, careful eating becomes not only synonymous with goodness, but also emerges as a practice through which one can embody goodness. This part therefore further unpacks the bio- and socio-political forces motivating careful eating.

The chapters further expose how discourses of careful food are entangled with a series of imaginaries or signified places – distanced and connected – as well as a rhetoric of the alternative, which together cohere to assemble and determine what constitutes careful, safe and socially responsible behaviour around eating. Here, then, place(s), the good and the safe are shown to be intertwined, uniting as mutually informing potencies that compel, drive and influence food preferences. Associatively, real and imagined distances between eaters and what 'should' be eaten emerge as instrumental to enacting careful eating. Notions of proximity and distance are thereby demonstrated to be pivotal to how careful foods are conceptualized, with perceived disconnects from and around food production shown to strain and stretch how food is understood, embraced or rejected. Furthermore, distances enable foods to embed into socially acceptable narratives and new social places, thereby fashioning places from which to care from and in. As the chapters demonstrate, new technologies are also actively supporting the emergence of these (imagined) geographies of careful eating. As such, strangers deliver webs of anonymous (cyber)care, distances are transformed into proximities, and carers, eater and foods become 'connected'.

Chapter 7

Placing Security: Food, Geographical Knowledge(s) and the Reproduction of Place(less-ness)

Benjamin Coles

Food Security and Securing Food: A Geographer's Perspective

One of the more profound shifts in contemporary food provision is consumers and producers variously seeking to reclaim food from agri-industrial capitalism. This shift has most typically been sited within a range of 'alternative' food networks and initiatives that articulate an array of ethics surrounding consumption and production. As such, it suggests that likeminded consumers and producers (and a host of interconnected actors within food provision more broadly) increasingly care about food and the modes, methods and ultimately places that are implicated in its production, processing, retail and consumption. Along with this shift, various agents increasingly demonstrate a concern to secure food from what they perceive to be systems that reject the inequities, imbalances and injustices of agri-industrial food methods. By engaging with, and explicitly acknowledging, the geographies and geographical relations that underscore these efforts to secure food, their actions demonstrate the extent to which they care about food and the spaces and places from which it emerges.

This chapter considers what happens to spaces and places when food is framed by entangled notions of security and care. It does this using the example of Fred and Ginger, an affluent, mixed-race couple from London who claim they care about the food they eat and use this caring to inform their consumption. The pseudonyms, which were chosen by the couple to signify comedic Hollywood actors and renowned dance partners Fred Astaire and Ginger Rogers, take on particular, though perhaps unknown (to Fred and Ginger), resonances within this account. In a comment attributed to former Whitehouse staff member Faith Wittlesey and appropriated by former Texas Governor Ann Richards (in a speech at the 1988 Democratic Convention), it was said that Ginger Rogers did everything that Fred Astaire did, only backwards and in heels. In the account I give here, Ginger does quite a lot of the work when it comes to food provision and caring. As a couple, Ginger and Fred are an indicative (rather than representative) example, whom I present in order to provoke broader questions about food, consumption and practices that surround security and care – practices that, as the other contributions to this volume demonstrate, are themselves multiple and partial. Taking this perspective, this chapter thus confronts the contradictions and paradoxes that emerge in association with one form of caring about food, and, in the process, explores the other spaces that are produced when food is secured.

Owing to a range of 'asymmetric threats best represented by concerns for climate change, peak oil and financial turmoil' (Sage 2014: 255), contemporary food provision is often cast as 'insecure' (Bohle et al. 1994; Brown and Funk 2008; Lang and Heasman 2004). Furthermore, such insecurity is typically projected onto the 'folk devil' (see Jackson 2010) of 'conventional', 'global' agri-capitalism, and the seemingly inherent inequities that come along with a food system in which profit-seeking is the organizing principle. Through the state's participation in global commodity exchange and its compliance with international regulation and governance (Jarosz 2011), it ensures that enough food is made available to feed its population and that this is safe from pathogens, contamination and adulteration. The latter also posits food security into audit-based regulatory frameworks that help to detect threats and identify liability when things go wrong (Dunn 2007). Thus, food security is both about feeding people and ensuring the free movement of materials in order to reproduce the political economic function of the state. Crucially, food security becomes enmeshed with broader regulatory security regimes (see Dikeç 2013) with remits that range from the capacity to mitigate fraud to the power to secure borders and control the movement of bodies.

Security implies a space free from care, worry or anxiety (Coles 2013). When it comes to food it means not only having enough food, but also having enough of the right kind of food. It also means not having to worry about these types of food issues – in effect, not having to care about food. As a spatial practice, security delineates the safe from the unsafe and the self from the Other. A state of security in essence frees the self from having to be concerned with Others by demarcating the spaces in which Others, and the hazards they embody, can be safely deposited, and by policing the borders of such spaces. These spatial configurations that secure self from Other are evident in prisons (see Sibley and Van Hoven 2009), gated communities (see Low 2001), or indeed as I touch upon later, the *banlieues* of suburban France (see Dikeç 2008), as well as in the everyday ideological assemblages that frame an array of class-based, ethnic, gendered and/or racialized politics. Security thus implies a political process that identifies hazards, territorializes differences and excludes them from space and place.

When it comes to discourse and debate around food, spaces of security and insecurity are activated through multiple scales, spaces and materialities. Food security is often tied to the big questions of gross national production and distribution, conditions of abject poverty and concerns over net caloric intake, and the ability of states to generate enough capital to feed their populations. Food security is thereby often thought of a national problem, an issue for poor countries – particularly those in the global south – and it is addressed through increased production, international trade, aid, accord and goodwill (Clapp 2012; McDonald 2010). In this context, and at this scale, food security can also become a state tool for the subjugation and control of populations (Nally 2008; Nally 2011), as well as a space of resistance, struggle and emancipatory potential (Heynen 2009, 2010; Heynen et al. 2012; Wilson 2013).

Food security is also a technological problem, particularly from the perspective(s) of biosecurity, which secures food from infectious and hazardous agents. Employing a complex array of actors, technologies and modes of governance, this type of security seeks to maintain bio-secure, safe spaces and, in the process, attempts to exclude actual and perceived threats. The purpose of such security is twofold; it seeks both to secure space by ensuring that pathogens do not contaminate the food supply, and also to secure economic function within a neoliberal food regime by facilitating the trade of foodstuffs throughout an international food system (Hinchliffe et al. 2013; Hinchliffe and Bingham 2008; Maye et al. 2012; Pechlaner and Otero 2010). Security, in this sense, is constituted through specific discursive practices that assemble a multiplicity of local sites to respond to particular events in which biosecurity is threatened, breached or has failed (Everts 2013). Food biosecurity becomes interlinked with notions of geopolitical food security through an array of market devices and governance stratagems in which states and international bodies collaborate in the production and distribution of foodstuffs and come together to delineate secure spaces that protect and ensure the security of food – for the health and safety of populations (or their control) and to maintain trade as part of a neoliberal market-based food economy (Busch 2010).

At the consumption level, however, efforts to secure food fall out of these systemic regulatory regimes and instead range from day-to-day struggles to afford and procure the body's basic reproductive needs (see Dowler et al. 2011; Kneafsey et al. 2013) to more nuanced forms of cultural reproduction in which food is secured from an affective register of socially reproduced anxieties (Milne et al. 2011; Jackson 2010). My focus here, however, is on end-consumers, such as Ginger and Fred, who are otherwise subjected to security's top-down technological measures. I am interested in the ways in which they incorporate perspectives on security and fold them into their own praxes of care and caring. Along the way, such consumers reproduce their own secure spaces and adapt them to variously reclaim or otherwise 'secure' food from what they perceive to be its 'insecurities'. Particularly, I focus on the ways in which end-consumers employ geographical narratives, specifically discourses of place (and place-making), to secure their foods from the inequities and insecurities that characterise the agri-capitalist food system and ensure that their food supply is free from cares, worries and anxieties. Morgan (2010), focusing particularly on the exploration of 'alternative food' – foods that simultaneously highlight insecurity and seek to mitigate it – suggests food is 'the ultimate index of our capacity to care for ourselves and for others, be they our 'nearest and dearest' or 'distant strangers': he notes that food plays a 'unique role in human reproduction, shaping our physical and cognitive development', and that without it, 'human life is "nasty, brutish and short"' (ibid.: 1852). Through this perspective, we see that food, security and care are interrelated and are made visible by consumers in the ways they articulate a range of concerns about personal and family health, other people, animals and the environment. The practices of consumption shaped by such concerns 'place' and 're-place' foods into a palatable imaginative geography of safe and, by extension, unsafe spaces and places.

Alternative foods typically deploy a range of place narratives to highlight such imaginative geographies as ways to distinguish themselves from what is otherwise described as a 'placeless foodscape' (Holloway and Kneafsey 2000). Place is the frame through which people conceptualize and interact with the world around them (Sack 1992, 2001a; Tuan 1974). It is also the site onto which geographical imaginations – the ability to envision geographical connection – and imaginative geographies – the representations of those connections – are founded. Contemporary food provision is rife with such geographies that appear through various celebrations, narratives, 'knowledges' and representations of place and placeless-ness, and consumers are complicit in their reproduction (Coles and Crang 2011; Cook and Crang 1996). Subsequently, owing to the wide assortment of places in which consumers engage with food, the ways places are assembled matter to how consumers experience food and conceptualize their consumption. This chapter demonstrates that the ways in which consumers articulate their practices of care and security map closely onto the discourses of 'knowledges' and visibilities that have come to be associated with alternative foods. Indeed, perceived visibility and invisibility play important roles in shaping how consumers 'see' their consumption, whilst place and place-making are central to how consumers enact their consumption.

Methodologically, as well as conceptually, this chapter is broadly topographic (Coles 2014). It is informed empirically by a long-term, multi-sited research programme comprised of structured and semi-structured interviews, informal chats, participant observation, site-writing, photography and archival research in and on an array of locales associated with food provision: street markets, supermarkets, farms, households and kitchens, abattoirs, corporate boardrooms and a host of other-such known and unknown, imagined and real places, whose interrelatedness make-up a geography of contemporary food provision. The aim of such topography in general is to articulate and analyse the role of place and place-making in the constitution of food provisioning practices, Particular to this chapter and volume, the aim of the two topographic cuts presented is to highlight how the partiality of any one place and perspective within food provision (or indeed foods' geographies more broadly), such as Ginger and Fred's, can be mobilized to tease out other questions about foods' consumption and its geographies, such as those around security or care.

Using the seeming ubiquity of chicken as a starting point, this chapter explores the dynamics between care and caring, security and securing, and place and place-making across Southeast London. I examine the ways in which Ginger and Fred, who reside in Camberwell, South London, deploy place to both secure food and to demonstrate that they care about it and its geographies. Ginger and Fred are affluent London barristers who identify themselves as high-investors into the ideologies that underlie alternative food. They express concern for their own health and wellbeing, as well as those of the environment, people and animals that make up the food system, stating that they 'care about their food, where it comes from and all of the things that goes along with that'. They both buy and buy into arguments that food should be produced as locally as possible, and tell me that 'we as consumers should support British farming', which also entangles the politics of care with those of class, ethnicity and nationalism. Fred and Ginger maintain that they focus their consumption on alternative and otherwise 'ethical' foods, shopping in 'local' markets for some items and 'organic' butchers for others, but also, primarily, through the web-based delivery service, Ocado. Furthermore as barristers who routinely work irregular hours, they also incorporate a range of other practices into their provisioning strategies ranging, as Fred puts it, 'from the dodgy Chinese take away down the street, where you don't know what kind of meat you are eating, to train station sandwiches with chicken from anywhere, to a proper Sunday roast'. Fred and Ginger's perspective is not representative of the other consumers with whom I have worked over the course of this programme *per se*. However, their perspectives on and anxieties around food consumption, as well as attempts to utilize their consumption to address the multivalent contradictions presented within contemporary food, resonate across a broader spectrum of agents, discourses and places within food.

Chickens and Camberwell

Chickens represent a critical fulcrum in this discussion about the relationship between care and security, and about how consumers use narratives of place to reclaim and secure food from the placeless foodscape of contemporary agri-capitalism. The spatial contradictions and paradoxes that I signalled earlier materialize in the bodies of these modern chickens and the ways in which they are consumed. The modern broiler chicken stereotypically embodies and reflects notions of an uncaring food landscape – a place in which the birds are stripped of their identity by a techno-science and economic assemblage designed to reduce sentient beings into 'crops' – and subsequently re-think them in terms of 'yields', 'cycles' and 'production times'. Indeed, nearly all chickens that we eat in the global north and west are the (bi)products of our agri-industrial food complex (see Boyd and Watts 1997; Buller and Roe 2014; Godley and Williams 2009). Fashioned through research and development, corporate agri-business and shifting social and economic policy, the modern broiler chicken is actually a very successful bi-product of the egg industry. Their scales of production reflect that success: '[T]here are some 17 billion domestic chickens worldwide, being equivalent to a ratio of 2.5 of these birds for every human (FAO 2007). There are approximately 29 million laying hens and 116 million broilers in the UK at any one time' (DEFRA 2010: 3). Nearly all these chickens are from the seemingly placeless foodscape and they occupy some of the more troubling spaces within it, including high-density production facilities, and extremely high-capacity slaughterhouses. As a result, their bodies become primary sites onto which the regimes of bio and geo-political security are projected, and which have the potential to represent a serious threat to food security and world health at large (Lowe 2010).

Camberwell, like the rest of London and other cities and towns, contains a cosmopolitan foodscape in which consumers can opt in or out of an array of placed and placeless foods in order to secure food, and in the process draw their own boundaries around what is safe and unsafe (to eat). It is a rapidly gentrifying, up and coming neighbourhood in South London and is at the confluence of a variety of competing and often-contradictory food-sheds. There are local farmers' markets, and other sites and opportunities to consume foods that align with typical alternative narratives of place, provenance and so-called good food.[1] There is also a range of ethnic and ethnicized food outlets such as grocers, supermarkets and restaurants that, to varying degrees, highlight food provenances in which material authenticity rather than alternative food's placed narratives are channelled. There are also other local markets, fruit and vegetable vendors, butchers and miscellaneous food purveyors in which narratives of place/alternative take a backseat to other qualities, such as convenience, ethnicity, and or price. Flanked by affluent Dulwich on one side and more deprived Peckham on the other, Camberwell functions as a security 'borderland' in which multiple spaces of security and insecurity are enacted and come together (see Hincliffe et al. 2013).

Ocado: Chickens in Camberwell

According to the information on the packet of the first chicken I want to discuss, it is 'free range', 'organic' and produced by 'selected British farms'. The packet arrives in Camberwell at Ginger and Fred's house in the back of an Ocado delivery van. Ocado is an online supermarket that allows customers to order deliveries either from their website or through a smartphone app that enables customers to browse goods, place them in a 'trolley' and 'checkout'. The packet's label is blue and green, with a Union Jack in the top right corner, and text and images on the front. The text includes preparation and storage advice orientated around biosecurity, e.g. washing hands, keeping refrigerated, cooking to an adequate temperature (to kill bacteria such as campylobacter), and nutrition information, e.g. calories, protein, sugar and fat. It also contains a geographical narrative about chicken production and a line drawing of two chickens scratching around on the ground. The narrative text reads:

> Our organic chickens are reared exclusively for Waitrose on small, organically-
> certified farms in Northern Ireland. By day they are free to roam in open pastures

---

1   Gibson-Graham (2014) provides a list of key buzzwords that are used to describe notions of 'alternative' economies from which the discourses of alternative foods are typically derived.

and exhibit their natural behaviour. By night, they are protected in purpose built sheds and are fed an organic cereal based diet.

This text and image together evoke the familiar, albeit ambiguous, language and landscape of 'good food' (Sage 2003). The explicit references to 'small farms', 'open pastures', being 'free to roam' and 'natural behaviour' provide Fred and Ginger with a geographical imaginary that mobilizes a range of tropes associated with alternative and good food movements. This imaginary, when juxtaposed with blank packets of chicken without evocative descriptions, fashions an image of what the spaces of chicken production ought to be like, whilst also fashioning an image of what they ought not to be like. The former, according to the packet, is procured from Waitrose and makes further branding associations between Waitrose and a general sense of goodness within their foods. The latter refers, presumably, to their competition and associates it with whatever the opposite spaces of good food might be – bad food. Sage (2003: 51) posits good food as a 'dialectical alternative' to the bad foods produced 'without due consideration of the naturalness, provenance and quality of its ingredients, food which has not been produced with the highest regard for animal welfare, the environment and the nutritional well-being of its consumers' (see also Maye et al. 2007).

According to Ginger, she cares about:

> ...the people who grow food...even the animals. If they've [the animals] had a happy life, I feel better about it because it probably means they've been looked after and are safer...I feel really strongly about it when it comes to chickens...I read something or saw a documentary about battery chickens and how horrible is that? That's why we only eat free range and organic chickens...

Ginger draws a connection between good animal husbandry practices (in her words animals that have been 'looked after') and food safety. To extrapolate, for Ginger *caring* about production (e.g. free range, and/or organic chicken farming, etc), leads to at least some notion of safer, better food. While Ginger and Fred both comment that they care that the chickens they eat are allowed to roam and be natural in a protective environment, they also reveal that they (in their words) 'prefer British chickens' because they are 'safer', more secure and 'more ethical' than chickens from 'other countries like Brazil'. Notions of safety and security become bound-up in both husbandry practices and also a nationalist discourse that places good within the UK and places bad in an Othered foreign foodscape.

The modern broiler chicken, however, regardless of how it has been farmed – whether it is organic, free range, or raised in a barn, or indeed grown in the UK or anywhere else – bears little resemblance to the 'natural' chicken evoked by the packet from which Ginger and Fred consume. Instead it is produced through a techno-scientific assembly of genetic manipulation (of both chicken bodies and feed) that prioritizes particular features of the chicken's body, such as larger breasts for white meat, and particular attributes of a chicken's life – specifically compressing the time from hatching to slaughter into as few weeks as possible, and this is true for all chickens in a supermarket (see Striffler 2005; Stull and Broadway 2013). Additionally, modern chickens are produced through a system of industrialized cropping and contract farming, and ultimately large-scale slaughter, processing and packaging (see Boyd and Watts 1997). This, in turn, is only made possible through extensive, carbon-intensive systems of cold-chains, supermarket market consolidation, and centralized distribution that reduces the individuality of the animal into a crop (Buller 2013; Godley and Williams 2009). When questioned, however, neither Ginger nor Fred is aware of these materialities. Instead, they have to rely on the descriptors on the packet. Ginger, who identifies herself as 'anxious' about what she eats, is desperate for information about, as she puts it, 'the realities of food' and turns to me with her questions, 'it's [organic/free range chicken] got to be better, right?'.

Narratives like the one on the packet connect consumers with imagined materialities of food production that ultimately cannot exist within the ways in which contemporary food provision is organized, nor within the ways that Fred and Ginger procure food. Rather, these narratives entangle food into a double fetish that deploys geographical knowledges to illuminate an imaginary of production, further obscures its materialities and insulates consumers from these materialities. Ginger's knowledge of chicken production plays into a configuration that, in her words, produces 'safe' 'happy' British chickens, conflates these ideas with technical implications of 'free range' and 'organic', and juxtaposes them with the perceived horrors of 'battery' chicken farming from abroad. The result is that even though they are suspicious of supermarket practices (as discussed below), Ginger and Fred are willing to accept narratives on the package, if not as truth then at least as a proxy for greater equity in food. I argue, however, that as Ginger and Fred buy into such narratives, they simultaneously reinforce inherent and problematic binaries of happy and unhappy and of organic/free-range and 'battery' chickens. These narratives therefore contribute to putting practices into play that maintain the dualities that characterize contemporary food provision and further normalize the spaces of bad and good food whilst appearing to challenge them.

Fred and Ginger use the stories on packets to place their consumption within a food landscape/imaginary they care about. Likewise, they are aware of the limitations of such stories. They are aware that the landscape portrayed through the text and imagery on the packet, although factually accurate, may bear little resemblance to commercial chicken farms, where the two artfully-rendered birds pecking around a farmyard will be surrounded by thousands of others (Lowry and Miele 2011). They are aware that the packaging does not signal the complexity of chicken farming; either its history or the current system of contract farms, centralized production controls, and the other elements that characterize modern food production.

Ginger and Fred are less aware, however, of the label and packaging's broader implications. By flagging its own food spaces as good, the packaging tacitly acknowledges the ethically and morally dubious practices that occur elsewhere within chicken farming. It places these practices, however, onto Other producers and retailers that subscribe to them. This suggestion is made by constructing an image through labelling and other geographical representations that counters the imagined images of battery chicken farms and industrial meat production at large – the images that shape Ginger's, in particular, understanding of food production. The packaging, more significantly, fixes the image of 'good food' production and normalizes it within a specific spatial imaginary: one of pastures and freedom, and healthy, happy, natural animals. The effect of this good food space is twofold: it reinforces the idea that unhappy, unhealthy animals also exist but that they are locked away in some other space. But more problematically, it also normalizes images of good food and, by extension, what caring about good food might entail and how these cares might be enacted – namely through a particular kind of consumption (see Abbots and Coles 2013).

What I find fascinating about this first cut is that, in locating the source of their food, Ginger and Fred demonstrate their caring about food; in locating its production methods, its geographies become visible and appear secure. Paradoxically, as this happens, the rest of the process simultaneously dis/appears within the placeless realms of the neoliberal food regime(s) (Campbell 2009; Pechlaner and Otero 2010). Fred and Ginger's placed chicken arrives already processed into small parts and ready to be consumed. It emerges from the inside of a van and, upon scanning, it figuratively, if not literally, leaves Ocado's network of inventory control where it was a unit with a barcode (Dodge and Kitchin 2004). Before arriving at Ocado, the chicken was slaughtered, butchered and packaged, yet the places in which these processes happen remain obfuscated. When pressed, Ginger and Fred are aware that these places must exist, but they are distanced from them, the ethical challenges they might present, and the moral imperatives to act that come with a more complete geographical awareness (Sack 2001b).

Hanging Chickens, 'Safe' Chickens

> When we have time, we go to the good butcher... he knows what he's talking about...he's not like the supermarkets who are just out there to make money...I feel better about going to the butcher, and buying his meat (Fred).

On their website, this butcher states:

> Our main suppliers of beef are [X] who mature their beef traditionally on the bone and [Y] [from] Lakenheath in Suffolk who specialise [sic] in pedigree rare breed beef. In pork we have welfare friendly Suffolk pork from [Z]. We now stock [W] free range chicken, where happy birds taste better as well as organic free range [V] chickens, a treasure from Suffolk.

For Ginger and Fred, this is what a caring food landscape consists of: not only high-welfare, but also 'pedigree' 'rare breed' animals that appear in the butcher's display as somehow not subsumed into an undifferentiated corporate industrial foodscape. In addition, and crucially, these qualities of care ultimately lead, according to the butcher, to better tasting food – a proposition that Fred and Ginger support. Referencing specific places of production suggests that narratives of place, and caring about places, matter to consumers. At the same time, however, it does not matter to consumers, such as Fred and Ginger, what places get evoked, whether it is somewhere in Suffolk, or any number of other places that produce the kind of food that stock the butcher's counter, so long as they conform to a shared understanding of 'good food' spaces, and so long as the food does indeed come from some specific, however imagined, place – in this case, 'Suffolk' with its 'good tasting', 'happy birds', 'welfare friendly' pork and 'traditional' 'pedigree', 'rare-breed beef', and indeed Dulwich, where the good butcher resides. For Fred and Ginger, this butcher in Dulwich and other similarly positioned food purveyors who deploy such discourses and imaginaries help to reproduce their image of a placed food landscape, one that is safe and secure so long as its geographies are identifiable and maintained. The attention paid to provenance and tradition, whilst also ensuring welfare, presumably means that these food stuffs are 'good to eat', and 'good' for a number of other reasons (Goodman et al. 2010).

What they do not buy through Ocado, or the good butcher, Fred and Ginger purchase locally: the delis, the multiple ethnic grocers and other such purveyors that make up Camberwell's food landscape. 'Local' for them, however, must still conform to idealized spaces that fit into these geographical imaginaries of good food.

> This butcher [the 'good butcher' in Dulwich] has good quality meat, not like those ones that we saw on Peckham High Street…you don't know where that meat comes from…it could be anywhere. Not all of it's expensive at the butcher though…I also feel strongly about supporting British farmers. And in Dulwich, everything is British, and is organic…' (Ginger).

They do not buy meat in Peckham, which is closer and therefore more local than Dulwich. They only go there to catch trains, for a *flâneur* experience in the market or on the high street, the odd trip to a Persian themed spice shop, or because Ginger 'can't help buying household stuff like dishwasher tablets or laundry detergent …[at] the pound shop'.

Rye Lane, one of Peckham's main shopping streets is a ten minute walk from Fred and Ginger's house. Dulwich, where the good butcher is, is a bit further away. During one of our sessions, we went to Peckham as part of their 'Saturday morning routine'. As usual for the couple, this includes a late breakfast at one of the nearby cafés that appeal to Camberwell's emergent foodie culture by serving single origin coffee and 'artisan' pastries – and a trip to a spice shop on Peckham Road before heading to a refurbished pub to read the papers and chat. Peckham is characterized as a poor inner city borough of London comprising migrant and working class populations, but one that on the surface is socially mixed and appears to celebrate 'happy multiculturalism' (see Ahmed 2010). As Jackson and Benson (2014: 1201 quoting Butler and Robson 2001: 78) note, however, Peckham is also marked by 'tectonic' relations, where 'social groups or 'plates' overlap or run parallel to one another without much in the way of integrated experience in the areas' social and cultural institutions'.

Rye Lane is lined with small shops and numerous butchers and fishmongers catering to both the local diaspora and its working class population. Unlike the more upmarket butcher's in Dulwich, those in Peckham offer 'worryingly [to Ginger] inexpensive meat' – much of which is on display in conditions that Ginger is unsure of. Dead chickens and the odd duck hang in the windows – some have yet to be plucked, the odd fly buzzes around, the gutter is littered with rubbish, and there are odours not only of raw meat but raw meat near (or past) its prime and old fish.

The people in the butchers, both patrons and workers, are not as identifiably middle class as those who inhabit the 'good butcher' in Dulwich. Signage around the products signals the bargains that are available, particularly in comparison to the nearby 'Big 3' supermarkets. The products themselves – an array of meat (especially mutton and goat, poultry and fish not found in typical UK vendors [see Coles and Hallet 2012]); familiar and unfamiliar (to Ginger and Fred) fruit and vegetables; and a wide variety of packaged foodstuffs with labels in languages other than English – are indicative of the multi-classed, multi-racial, multi-ethnic food spaces in this area (Lyon and Back 2012). The pricing, however, indicates that these shops are aimed towards lower social economic groups, which for Ginger, who uses the price of meat as a marker for quality, also positions these shops as low quality. Ginger speculates that 'some of these butchers must also supply the local kebab shops… where you don't know what you're getting'. Beyond languages on the labels there does not appear to be any other mention of provenance. Labels that claim products to be free range, organic or otherwise produced with these ideals in mind are not evident, suggesting that food here is sold based on their material and utilitarian properties and demand (e.g. for ingredients for the variety of dishes that represent the tastes of nearby community members), as well as price, as opposed to other qualities relating to welfare, sustainability and other issues that Ginger and Fred care about (cf. Harvey et al. 2004).

This results in distinct food spaces for Fred and Ginger, the secure one that they inhabit and use to practise their politics of care and caring, and the Other one from which they demarcate their spaces of security. I must stress here that although Fred and Ginger are a mixed-race couple, except in helping to delineate various Other consumptive spaces that brush against each other but seldom overlap with Ginger and Fred's, questions of race and ethnicity are less important in informing their consumption than questions of affluence and class. As Jackson and Benson (2014: 1201) comment, Rye Lane, which provides people like Ginger and Fred with the opportunity to visually consume the Other from a position of security, bifurcates 'two worlds marked by ethnic and social difference': Fred and Ginger's 'world' juxtaposes middle class notions of security with the consumption (but not ingestion) of exotic dangers and the lived world of Others.

Care and caring are constructive processes. In order for Fred and Ginger to demonstrate that they care about their food, they must fashion its geographies. One geography imagines a food landscape of richly embedded social relations, high animal welfare, and a host of other positive associations and relationships around food production and consumption. This geography bypasses some of the messier places and spaces of food, such as slaughterhouses and meat packers, and is thus a partial representation of a caring food landscape (albeit one that only really exists in an imaginative form). The other geography is one of threats, dangers and Others comprised of unknown food and food origins, viscerally shocking displays and a sense of foreignness – either of Brazilian chickens or various other, non-British foodstuffs. Fred and Ginger's geography of care, in other words, fashions a geography to care about.

A tension, however, emerges between 'knowing' and 'knowledges'. The Dulwich butcher presents a sanitized version of meat production. Although it makes claims towards provenance and signals taste, pedigree and tradition, it brings Ginger and Fred no closer to the materialities of production than the packet of chicken from Ocado, or indeed the supermarket meat that Fred eschews. Ironically, the materialities that would bring the couple closer to production, such as the obviously dead, but not-quite meat, not-quite-plucked chickens in the butchers' windows in Peckham, provoke a sense of danger and disgust and are subsequently dismissed. They are perhaps too close to the realities of meat production, as well as located in seemingly unsafe spaces that are consumed visually, but no further. For consumers like Fred and Ginger, there is a desire to get closer to the imagined materialities of food production, but in a distanced, clean and safe manner. Food realities are messier, and evoke both feelings of disgust and insecurity and danger (see Abbots 2014; West 2014).

I am interested in the ways in which the visceral geographies of meat production that are presented in Peckham are refracted through sanitized narratives and secured in safe places like the Dulwich butcher. Ginger and Fred object to the materialities that might bring them closer to production and instead rely on imaginative geographical narratives that produce the illusion of proximity. Thus the illusion of being able to care is created for them, but this paradoxically also maintains, if not increases, the distances (and invisibilities) of their consumption. Where the supermarket (for Fred) is 'just out to make money' and the shops in Peckham are a 'bit too dodgy' – and only good for the mundane placeless purchasing of dishwasher tablets and hand sanitizer – the Dulwich butcher somehow fits between the two: offering enough of a geographical narrative to bring farms close enough to verify that their cares and anxieties are met, but far enough away not to disturb Ginger and Fred's sense of security.

Placing Security and Securing Place

Perceptions of visibility are vital components to the reproduction of secure spaces. Whilst its internal mechanisms remain opaque, the war on terror, perhaps the supreme example of security in a contemporary age, ensures that both its mission (to prevent terrorism) and its target (terrorism) remain highly visible, and this state of visibility is maintained through a security theatre of checkpoints, colour coded alerts and visible technologies of 'safety' and surveillance. Such security rests on the dichotomy between safe and unsafe spaces from which safety is wrought (Dikeç 2013; Ranciere 2004). Ginger and Fred operate within this dynamic of safe and unsafe in order to secure their food. By actively fashioning safe spaces they simultaneously fashion unsafe spaces in order to secure geographies that attend to their cares. These geographies reproduce so called 'sensible objects' that assemble into an ideology-reinforcing 'aesthetic regime' in which the need for security becomes normalized (Dikeç 2013; Ranciere 2004).

For Ginger, the images of 'battery' chickens and the well-documented ethical challenges that such chickens – and more generally contemporary food provision – present are superimposed onto the Othered spaces of Peckham's Rye Lane. These battery chickens, their images, their supposed (non-)places of production, and the discursive milieus in which they operate (particularly the ethical challenges they present) comprise one such distribution of 'sensible evidences' that justify Fred and Ginger's need to secure 'happy chickens' (and their geographies). Peckham too is constructed through images, media and popular representations as a space of danger associated with class and a related ethnic struggle, within which, as Blokland (2009) suggests, middle-class gentrifiers seek to claim and otherwise secure their own territories from these Others. In the words of Benson and Jackson (2013: 47), Peckham is a:

> loaded signifier, a place with a reputation...[associated] with a Cockney white working class...and with gang and gun crime...[but also] ... as a trendy, arty place...of (racialised) danger, an emerging cool art scene and an association with Trotters Independent Traders..

Battery chickens and Peckham combine into a threatening geography that presents an affront to the issues around food and the body that Ginger and Fred care about. For them, these geographies are largely unknown but are represented by placeless battery chicken farms and invisible connections that link these to 'dirty' butchers in 'dodgy' Peckham; there, chickens are not expensive enough to guarantee the safety, health and welfare standards that the couple care about. The two visions, of chickens and of Peckham, consolidate an aesthetic regime in which both become parts of the same insecure space. Ginger and Fred utilize this insecurity to justify their consumption practices. They reinforce their own secure spaces when they travel to Dulwich and when they purchase 'happy chickens' from Ocado, each of which emerges as a secure space through similar aesthetic assemblages.

This fashioning of security and insecurity, in turn, reproduces an ideology of security that has spatial consequences – namely that actual places are impacted by the consumption practices that Fred and Ginger employ. Place and place-making thus lies at the heart of this relationship between the secure and insecure. Regardless of what they are really like (if such a statement can stand), Peckham and battery chickens, and Dulwich and 'happy meat', are reproduced through co-constitutive imaginative geographical processes as much as they are through the material practices of consumption.

Sack (1992) suggests that all places of consumption hide their geographical interrelatedness – the awareness of which, he posits, inhibits the ability of consumers to make informed and for him intrinsically moral decisions (see also Sack 2003). Notions of geographical awareness underlie Fred and Ginger's concerns about health and wellbeing when it comes to food. I argue that this is why they go to the lengths they do to consume foods whose geographies are made seemingly apparent to them. Likewise, when these geographies remain invisible, they seek to consume narratives that 'place' them into a geography that fits their perceptions of safe and secure food. These visibilities allude to a geographical awareness that helps them to make sense of, and construct, places and geographies out of what is otherwise a placeless foodscape.

Towards a Moral Geography of Care and Security

Visible geographies are an important component in ensuring that food is secure from outside 'contaminants', be they pathogens, modes of unethical practice or close/distant Others that pose various threats to self-identity and society: 'Visibility is supposed to produce verity' (Dunn 2007: 49). Morgan (2010) suggests that 'alternative' food is one space in which a wide range of cares about people, animals and the environment come together, and where the connections lost to the placeless foodscape are reconnected – making it a space in which consumers can secure food from a food system whose very opaqueness makes it insecure. Conceptually, at least, alternative foods emerge from a tradition of alternative economies that, through their organization and practice, challenge the hegemony of contemporary neoliberal capitalism (Gibson-Graham 2006). For food, this tradition variously seeks to unravel and unveil the commodity fetish, in order reveal what Harvey (1990: 422) refers to as the 'fingerprints of exploitation' that underlie capitalist food production. Coles and Crang (2011) in an attempt to 'get with' commodity fetishism further argue that the appeal of alternative foods (and those that are positioned to appropriate the language and discourses of alternative foods) is that their geographies appear to be transparent and offer foodstuffs that do not fit into the conventional norms of agri-capitalism (see also Cook 2004; Cook and Crang 1996; Cook et al. 2004). They note that such foods come packaged in a range of semiotic devices and material culture, as well as testimony and testimonials, which posit them into a visible geography. They further note that place and place-making plays an important role in fashioning alternative foods. Not only do particular types of places become stages on which these visible geographies are performed – and subsequently consumed – they comprise didactic retail spaces that look, feel, and provide consumption experiences that are alternatives to more mundane forms of food provision.

Using these perspectives, I suggest that consumers, such as Ginger and Fred, buy into 'good' geographical narratives as a way to secure their own food consumption from that which is positioned as 'bad' and/or does not otherwise map onto good's discursive spaces (Goodman and Goodman 2007; Szasz 2007). When thinking about care it is easy to make ourselves believe that caring is a good thing; that it leads to better, more just, and indeed, 'good' outcomes because it not only raises awareness about the interconnections between the self and Others and between one place and others, but also seeks to produce more equitable relations between ourselves and Others, and ourselves and other places. Place, 'the frame on which the object, subject and intersubjective is founded' (Malpas 1999: 40), and place-making are central to this configuration, an argument that Larson and Johnson develop in their examination of affinity politics; in advocating an 'open sense of place', they conclude that such a sense:

> is guided by the recognition that situatedness is the singular motivating precondition for thought and action…sustained engagement with this place yields affinities that are…unpredictable and haphazard but also complementary to progressive political and moral praxis precisely because they are already attuned to humility and compassion (2012: 644).

Care and caring are thus bound to how place is conceived and activated.

When thinking about care and caring through the lens of consumption, however, it is possible to believe that these can be achieved (and demonstrated) by consuming – and leading others to consume – the right stuff. Particularly when it comes to foods that have been positioned as somehow alternative – and that subsequently slip into becoming somehow ethical – such consumption reveals the range of cares that are mobilized through food, its materialities and the places and spaces in which it is produced (and consumed). It is not too much of a stretch to then believe that such caring-through-consumption ultimately does good not only to the self, but to Others and to other places and that this sense of goodness emerges from the supposedly increased awareness of geographical interconnection and connectivity that careful consumption engenders. Additionally, it is possible to believe that caring not only secures food from a food system that, at least on the surface, appears to be rather uncaring, but also a broader range of individual, social, ecological and economic issues that are embedded into foods' materialities. Caring, I argue, is thus not only bound to the ways in which places and their interconnectivity are conceived and activated, but also to the ways in which they are articulated.

Care and caring through consumption, however, leads to spatial contradictions. They are performative acts of place that make free spaces – free from the worries, anxieties and cares that seemingly plague contemporary food provision. These spaces are secured through a range of practices that further reveal a multitude of concerns over contemporary food provision and their possible effects on bodies, societies, cultures and environments. But, these practices themselves mobilize processes that displace these concerns onto other spaces and thereby fashion them. Making one space secure requires making another insecure. This results in a contradiction in which care(s) becomes individualized, and secure spaces maintained through exclusion and exclusivity. Such consumption is ultimately predicated upon occluded geographies that proffer care to those who can afford it, and maintain it through regimes of isolated and marginalized spaces, which, when interrogated, reveal the very spatial unevenness that care is meant to resolve.

Fred and Ginger's story echoes that of nearly everyone I have talked with during the course of this project. They are interested in food, concerned about its production, willing to discuss how their cares translate into consumption practices, and, significantly, able to afford the increased production costs to which such cares ultimately lead. At the same time, they are broadly ignorant of the material realities (and the hidden spaces) that underlie food production, particularly of meat, as evidenced by Ginger turning to me for answers to assuage her self-labelled anxiety. Simply put, they have not been to the farms, abattoirs, factories and other such places that make up foods' geography and instead rely on an array of mediated representations of both good and bad food. The rub, however, is that even if their awareness were complete, which Sack (2004) argues is impossible, the ability to care, and also act, is contingent on a range of other factors – time and convenience being the main ones – but also a range of geographical knowledges about how places/spaces of food production interrelate with those of consumption. Fred and Ginger's story ultimately suggests how truly complex contemporary food provisioning really is, and how its multi-faceted layers are variously mediated through a range of fetishistic geographical narratives and imaginations about food's production spaces – narratives that both reveal and hide its materialities – and narratives about its spaces of consumption. The latter of these reveals that the cost of care and caring, through what always amount to partial perspectives, is the reproduction of exclusive spaces, the boundaries of which seem to be drawn along 'old' socio-geographic lines and speak to the broader questions of the inherent spatial-unevenness of capitalism (Smith 1984).

So, then what would an inclusive space of caring food look like within contemporary capitalism? Bringing this to a short conclusion, there is no such thing. The nature of capitalism necessitates winners and losers – whether people, spaces, or indeed animals. And, if notions of care are indeed mobilized through an array of fetishistic properties that join together places and spaces, imaginative geographies with bodies and materialities, care becomes morally fraught unless it is positioned first within a post-capitalist world in which such fetishes vanish.

Even then there is still the body of the chicken to contend with. Even 'happy' farmyard chickens have their throats cut.

References

Abbots, E-J. 2014. Embodying Country-City Relations: The Chola Cuencana in Highland Ecuador, in *Food Between the Country and the City: Ethnographies of a Changing Global Foodscape*, edited by N. Domingos, J.M. Sobral and H.G. West. London: Bloomsbury, 41-57.

Abbots, E-J. and Coles, B. 2013. Horsemeat-gate: The Discursive Production of a Neoliberal Food Scandal. *Food, Culture and Society: An International Journal of Multidisciplinary Research*, 16(4), 535-50.

Ahmed, S. 2010. *The Promise of Happiness*. Durham: Duke University Press.

Benson, M. and Jackson, E. 2013. Place-making and place maintenance: Performativity, place and belonging among the middle classes. *Sociology*, 47(4), 793-809.

Blokland, T. 2009. Celebrating local histories and defining neighbourhood communities: Place-making in a gentrified neighbourhood. *Urban Studies*, 46(8), 1593-610.

Bohle, H.G, Downing, T.E. and Watts, M.J. 1994. Climate change and social vulnerability: Toward a sociology and geography of food insecurity. *Global Environmental Change*, 4(1), 37-48.

Boyd, W. and Watts, M. 1997. The chicken industry and postwar American capitalism, in *Globalising Food: Agrarian Questions and Global Restructuring*, edited by D. Goo and M. Watts. London: Routledge, 139-64.

Brow, M.E. and Fun, C.C. 2008. Food security under climate change. *Science* 319(5863), 580-81.

Buller, H. 2013. Individuation, the mass and farm animals. *Theory, Culture & Society*, 30(7-8), 155-75.

Buller, H. and Roe, E. 2014. Modifying and commodifying farm animal welfare: The economisation of layer chickens. *Journal of Rural Studies*, 33, 141-9.

Busch, L. 2010. Can fairy tales come true? The surprising story of neoliberalism and world agriculture. *Sociologia Ruralis*, 50(4), 331-51.

Butler, T. and Robson, G. 2001. Social capital, gentrification and neighbourhood change in London: A comparison of three south London neighbourhoods. *Urban Studies*, 38(12), 2145-62.

Campbell, H. 2009. Breaking new ground in food regime theory: Corporate environmentalism, ecological feedbacks and the 'food from somewhere' regime? *Agriculture and Human Values*, 26(4), 309-19.

Clapp, J. 2012. *Hunger in the Balance: The New Politics of International Food Aid*. Ithaca, NY: Cornell University Press.

Coles, B. and Hallett, L. 2012. Eating from the bin: Salmon heads, waste and the markets that make them. *The Sociological Review*, 60(S2), 156-73.

Coles, B. and Crang, P. 2011. Placing alternative consumption: Commodity fetishism in Borough Fine Foods Market, London, in *Ethical Consumption: A Critical Introduction*, edited by E. Potter and T. Lewis. London: Routledge, 87-102.

Coles, B. 2014. Making the market place: A topography of Borough Market. London. *Cultural Geographies*, 21, 515-23.

Coles, B. 2013b. Security in *Food Words: Essays in Culinary Culture*, edited by P. Jackson and the Conanx Group. London: Bloomsbury, 193-4.

Cook, I. 2004. Follow the thing: Papaya. *Antipode*, 36(4), 21.

Cook, I. and Crang, P. 1996. The world on a plate. *Journal of Material Culture*, 1(2), 131-53.

Cook, I., Crang, P. and Thorpe, M. 2004. Tropics of consumption: 'getting with the fetish' of 'exotic' fruit?, in *Geographies of Commodity Chains*, edited by A. Hughes and S. Reimer. Abingdon: Routledge, 173-92.

DEFRA 2010. *Poultry in the United Kingdom: The Genetic Resources of the National Flocks*. London: DEFRA Report PB13451.

Dikeç, M. 2008. *Badlands of the Republic: Space, Politics and Urban Policy*. Oxford: Blackwell.

Dikeç, M. 2013. Immigrants, banlieues, and dangerous things: Ideology as an aesthetic affair. *Antipode*, 45(1), 23-42.

Dodge, M. and Kitchin, R. 2004. *Codes of Life: Identification Codes and the Machine-readable World* (CASA Working Papers 82). Centre for Advanced Spatial Analysis (UCL): London, 85-881.

Dowler, E.A., Kneafsey, M. Lambie H., Inman A. and Collier, R. 2011. Thinking about 'food security': Engaging with UK consumers. *Critical Public Health*, 21(4), 403-16.

Dunn, E. 2007. Escherichia coli, corporate discipline and the failure of the sewer state. *Space and Polity*, 11(1), 35-53.

Everts, J. 2013. Announcing swine flu and the interpretation of pandemic anxiety. *Antipode*, 45(4), 809-25.

FAO 2007. *The State of the World's Animal Genetic Resources for Food and Agriculture*, edited by B. Rischkowsky and D. Pilling. Rome. FAO Report.

Gibson-Graham, J.K. 2006. *A Postcapitalist Politics*. Minneapolis, MN: University of Minnesota Press.

Gibson-Graham, J.K. 2014. Rethinking the economy with thick description and weak theory. *Current Anthropology*, 55, S147-S153.

Godley, A. and Williams, B. 2009. Democratizing Luxury and the Contentious 'Invention of the Technological Chicken' in Britain. *Business History Review*, 83(2), 267-90.

Goodman, D. and Goodman, M. 2007. Localism, livelihoods, and the 'post-organic': Changing perspectives on alternative food networks in the United States, in *Alternative Food Geographies: Representation and Practice*, edited by D. Maye, L. Lewis and M. Kneafsey. Oxford: Elver, 23-38.

Goodman, M.K., Maye D. and Holloway, L. 2010. Ethical foodscapes?: Premises, promises, possibilities. *Environment and Planning A*, 42(8), 1782-96.

Harvey, D. 1990. Between space and time: Reflections on the geographical imagination. *Annals of the Association of American Geographers* 80(3), 418-34.

Harvey, M., McMeekin, A. and Warde, A. 2004. Introduction, in *Qualities of Food*, edited by M. Harvey, A. McMeekin and A. Warde. Manchester: Manchester University Press, 1-18.

Heynen, N. 2009. Bending the bars of empire from every ghetto for survival: The Black Panther Party's radical antihunger politics of social reproduction and scale. *Annals of the Association of American Geographers*, 99(2), 406-22.

Heynen, N. 2010. Cooking up non-violent civil-disobedient direct action for the hungry: 'Food not bombs' and the resurgence of radical democracy in the US. *Urban Studies*, 47(6), 1225-40.

Heynen, N., Kurtz, H.E. and Trauger, A. 2012. Food justice, hunger and the city. *Geography Compass*, 6(5), 304-11.

Hinchliffe, S. and Bingham, N. 2008. Securing life: The emerging practices of biosecurity. *Environment and Planning A*, 40(7), 1534-51.

Hinchliffe, S., Allen, J., Lavau, S., Bingham, N. and Carter, S. 2013. Biosecurity and the topologies of infected life: From borderlines to borderlands. *Transactions of the Institute of British Geographers*, 38(4), 531-43.

Holloway, L. and Kneafsey, M. 2000. Reading the space of the farmers' market: A preliminary investigation from the UK. *Sociologia Ruralis*, 40(3), 285-99.

Jackson, E. and Benson, M. 2014. Neither 'deepest, darkest Peckham' nor 'run-of-the-mill' East Dulwich: The middle classes and their 'Others' in an Inner-London neighbourhood. *International Journal of Urban and Regional Research*, 38(4), 1195-210.

Jackson, P. 2010. Food stories: Consumption in an age of anxiety. *Cultural Geographies*, 17(2), 147-65.

Jarosz, L. 2011. Defining world hunger: Scale and neoliberal ideology in international food security policy discourse. *Food, Culture and Society: An International Journal of Multidisciplinary Research*, 14(1), 117-39.

Kneafsey, M., Dowler, E., Lambie-Mumford, H Inman, A. and Collier, R. 2013. Consumers and food security: Uncertain or empowered? *Journal of Rural Studies*, 29 (January), 101-12.

Lang, T. and Heasman, M. 2004. *Food Wars: The Global Battle for Mouths, Minds and Markets*. London: Earthscan.

Larsen, S.C. and Johnson, J.T. 2012. Toward an open sense of place: phenomenology, affinity, and the question of being. *Annals of the Association of American Geographers*, 102(3), 632-46.

Low, S.M. 2001. The edge and the center: Gated communities and the discourse of urban fear. *American Anthropologist*, 103(1), 45-58.

Lowe, C. 2010. Viral clouds: Becoming H5N1 in Indonesia. *Cultural Anthropology*, 25(4), 625-49.

Lowry, E. and Miele, M. 2011. The taste of happiness: Free-range chicken. *Environment and Planning A*, 43, 2076-90.

Lyon, D. and Back, L. 2012. Fishmongers in a global economy: Craft and social relations on a London market. *Sociological Research Online*, 17(2), 23.

Malpas, J.E. 1999. *Place and Experience: A Philosophical Topography* Cambridge: Cambridge University Press.

Maye, D., Holloway, L. and Kneafsey, M. 2007. *Alternative Food Geographies: Representation and Practice*. Oxford: Elsevier.

Maye, D., Dibden, J., Higgins, V. and Potter, C. 2012. Governing biosecurity in a neoliberal world: Comparative perspectives from Australia and the United Kingdom. *Environment and Planning A*, 44, 150.

McDonald, B.L. 2010. *Food Security*. Cambridge: Polity.

Milne, R., Wenzer, J., Brembeck H. and Brodin, M. 2011. Fraught cuisine: Food scares and the modulation of anxieties. *Distinktion: Scandinavian Journal of Social Theory*, 12(2), 177-92.

Morgan, K. 2010. Local and green, global and fair: The ethical foodscape and the politics of care. *Environment and Planning A*, 42, 1852-67.

Nally, D. 2008. 'That coming storm': The Irish Poor Law, colonial biopolitics, and the Great Famine. *Annals of the Association of American Geographers*, 98(3), 714-41.

Nally, D. 2011, The biopolitics of food provisioning. *Transactions of the Institute of British Geographers*, 36, 37-53.

Pechlaner, G. and G. Otero. 2010, The neoliberal food regime: Neoregulation and the new division of labor in North America. *Rural Sociology*, 75(2), 179-208.

Ranciere, J. 2004. *The Politics of Aesthetics: The Distribution of the Sensible*. London: Continuum.

Sack, R. 1992. *Place, Modernity and the Consumer's World*. New York, NY: John Hopkins University Press.

Sack, R. 2001a. The geographic problematic: Empirical issues. *Norsk Geografisk Tidsskrif – Norwegian Journal of Geography*, 55(3), 107-16.

Sack, R. 2001b. The geographic problematic: Moral issues. *Norsk Geografisk Tidsskrif – Norwegian Journal of Geography*, 55(3), 117-25.

Sack, R. 2003. *A Geographical Guide to the Real and the Good*. London: Routledge.

Sage, C. 2003. Social embeddedness and relations of regard: Alternative 'good food' networks in south-west Ireland. *Journal of Rural Studies*, 19(1), 47-60.

Sage, C. 2014. The transition movement and food sovereignty: From local resilience to global engagement in food system transformation. *Journal of Consumer Culture*, 14(2), 254-75.

Sibley, D. and Van Hoven, B. 2009. The contamination of personal space: Boundary construction in a prison environment. *Area*, 41, 198-206.

Smith, N. 2008. *Uneven Development: Nature, Capital, and the Production of Space*. Athens, GA: University of Georgia Press.

Stull, D. and Broadway, M. 2013. *Slaughterhouse Blues: The Meat and Poultry Industry in North America*. Belmont, CA: Wadsworth Cengage Learning.

Striffler, S. 2005. *Chicken: The Dangerous Transformation of America's Favorite Food*. Yale, CT: Yale University Press.

Szasz, A. 2007. *Shopping Our Way to Safety: How We Changed From Protecting Our Environment to Protecting Ourselves*. Minneapolis, MN: University of Minnesota Press.

Tuan Y.F. 1974. *Topophelia: A Study of Environmental Perception, Attitudes and Values*. New York: Columbia University Press.

West, H. 2014. Bringing it all back home: Reconnecting the country and the city through heritage food tourism in the French Auvergne, in *Food Between the Country and the City: Ethnographies of a Changing Global Foodscape*, edited by N. Domingos, J Sobral and H.G West. London: Bloomsbury, 73-88.

Wilson, A.D. 2013. Beyond alternative: Exploring the potential for autonomous food spaces. *Antipode*, 45, 719-37.

Chapter 8

Configuring Relations of Care in an Online Consumer Protection Organization

Karin Eli, Amy K. McLennan and Tanja Schneider

Introduction

In this chapter, we explore tensions between expertise, care, and social responsibility enacted through and within HowToBuyWiki,[1] a Central European non-profit organization dedicated to the development of an emerging, open-source internet platform which, as the members describe it, is designed to promote 'product transparency'.[2] We draw on interviews carried out with HowToBuyWiki's six active members, as well as formal written records of their meetings and workshops, to examine the sometimes divergent ways in which care and authority take shape in the members' discourses of HowToBuyWiki's goals and methods, and their own positioning in the project. We pay particular attention to entanglements of responsibility, consumption, and care and, in so doing, highlight the ambiguities that inhere in this initiative to cultivate knowledgeable, caring, and careful consumer bodies. Specifically, we note the rhetorical and material roles of food in HowToBuyWiki's configurations of care, using the organization's discursive construction of chocolate on its wiki-platform as a case example.

---

1 HowToBuyWiki is a pseudonym. Throughout this chapter, we use 'group' or 'organization' to describe the HowToBuyWiki organizing committee, and 'member' to refer to each individually. People who consult the HowToBuyWiki website for information are referred to as 'users' or 'consumers', while those who add information are 'editors'. Users are generally not known to *HowToBuyWiki* members other than in the form of site-usage statistics and imagined identities; editors are recognized only by a self-selected pseudonym. 'Company' refers to an organization that produces and/or markets products; company representatives may also act as editors if they wish, and this is the case for several products listed on the wiki-platform.

2 As a result of the evolution of information and communication technologies (ICTs), there has been a continued rise in the number of wiki-style websites: platforms that permit users to share information collaboratively and dynamically, rather than passively view content. In 2009, one of the most famous of these, Wikipedia, was used as an information source by over 50 per cent of internet users (Reavley et al. 2013).

From May to October 2013, we[3] interviewed each of the six active committee members (hereafter members) of HowToBuyWiki (five in person, and one over Skype). The interviews were conducted with each member individually; while the interviews were semi-structured, and as such included overlapping questions, they also allowed each member to direct the conversation toward the issues and ideas most salient to her or his experience of the project. As the interview process unfolded, we found that HowToBuyWiki's story is one told through multiple, intersecting tensions. Through questions that called upon both actual and imagined experience, such as 'How did HowToBuyWiki start for you?', 'What would happen if users provided conflicting information?', and 'Who do you think HowToBuyWiki's users are?', the interviews delved into the members' dynamic framings of their project, which were entangled with negotiations of their own variable positioning as social entrepreneurs, leaders, knowledge brokers, and conscious consumers. In addition to the interviews, HowToBuyWiki provided us with access to website analytics, as well as to various documents, including the organization's constitution, student essays written about the platform, and archived meeting minutes, through which we could trace the development of HowToBuyWiki from its inception. We draw on all of these materials in this chapter.

Enabling Cyber-Care

Existing research has drawn attention to a multiplicity of ways in which care can be understood and practised (e.g. Thomas 1993; Mol et al. 2010). Care practices, according to Jespersen et al., 'involve both emotional and personal relationships as well as the ongoing inner workings of collectives' (2014: 666); here, care invokes attentiveness to others, whether they are individuals or communities, and responsiveness to them. Caregivers in US medical practice, for example, work with patients to 'decide how to balance the risks to the patient against the potential benefits to the same patient' (London and Kadane 2003: 62). Care practices in interventions for obesity trialled in Denmark involve combined collective efforts to alter dietary and exercise habits in ambiguous and messy collaborations between care providers and patients (Jespersen et al. 2014). Changes are not necessarily prescriptive, but are instead constantly negotiated and adjusted in an effort to achieve, where possible, both clinical improvement and patient satisfaction. Such interpersonal caring contrasts with other forms of care, such as governments' caring for their citizens, which are associated with political, legal and moral responsibility and authority (Tronto 1993; Williams 1995), and where care is determined and prescribed according to culturally-embedded notions of the 'right' and the 'good' (Barnes 2012).

---

3   The first author interviewed all six participants; the third author joined as co-interviewer in two of the six interviews; the second author transcribed all interviews verbatim.

Situated between interpersonal and authoritative care is the landscape of citizen-led care initiatives. Of particular salience to this chapter is community action for 'political consumerism' (Balsiger 2013), a form of informed consumption where citizens make 'choices among producers and products with the goal of changing objectionable institutional or market practices' (Micheletti 2003: 2). While most studies on political consumerism have focused on individual consumers, more recent work has begun to explore social movement organizations as pivotal agents, mobilizing consumers toward particular, politically-informed, modes of consumption (Forno and Graziano 2014: 140). Forno and Graziano suggest that Sustainable Community Movement Organizations (SCMOs) promoting political consumerism can be classified within a matrix, according to their '*attitude towards consumption*' (alter- or anti-) and '*predominant scale of action*' (local or global) (2014: 154, emphasis in original). The use of information and communication technologies (ICTs) as a primary mode of social action, however, complicates the latter part of this proposed typology. As Parigi and Gong argue, 'digital ties' (2014: 250), operate identically to face-to-face ties, and hence strengthen participation and commitment to the movement's cause, thus blurring the lines between local and global action. Likewise, Forno and Graziano argue that successful boycotts initiated via the internet have resulted in 'transnational awareness to step up pressure on corporations' and 'a broader sense of community' (2014: 141). Essential to such awareness and sense of community is the active forging of bonds of mutual solidarity and cooperation facilitated through the immediacy of social networking on the Internet (Lacey 2005). Perhaps the most prominent examples are the 2011 Arab Spring and Occupy protests: citizen-led political initiatives that amassed popular support through social media – and where, as Sutton et al. (2013) note, outrage over food prices and commodization, among other issues, played a catalyzing role.

While globalization and technical development may increase the global visibility of a cause, they may also influence how social movement organizations conceptualize and enact community-level and interpersonal care. HowToBuyWiki provides an example of a novel form of care that is facilitated by Internet-based technologies. Although HowToBuyWiki's members do not explicitly define their organization's practices as 'care', their emphasis on attending to ethical consumption issues, providing a responsive forum for consumer concerns, and promoting responsible (or 'conscious') consumption via a dedicated user community qualifies their practices as caring (as described by Jespersen et al. 2014; Thomas 1993) across the micro and macro levels. Mediated through words on a screen, the relationships they (aim to) develop are overlaid with ambiguity: users are imagined and yet remain anonymous; they interact and yet never encounter each other; they are provided with a platform for negotiation and personalization of data, yet must share knowledge in a rigid framework that limits their options and choices in order to (ostensibly) care for them.

Interwoven with the configuration of HowToBuyWiki's implicit objective of cyber-care is the negotiation of the *authority to care*. HowToBuyWiki offers more than an online platform to enact and reproduce already-extant relationships of care.

Placing community participation and a re-structuring of knowledge at its core, HowToBuyWiki is situated to create new dynamics that blur the directionality of expertise and care. Like other wiki platforms, HowToBuyWiki adheres to a governance structure which relies on community-building, user expertise, and an ethic of altruism and mutual responsibility. Each user, then, is invested with the responsibility to provide and accept care in the form of community expertise. In practice, however, as this chapter will show, HowToBuyWiki negotiates the multiple loci of expertise, and the multi-directionality of care they entail, through assuming primary responsibility for the enabling of cyber-care.

While HowToBuyWiki configures cyber-care as (enabling) the sharing of information on consumer products online, the organization's own relations of care are centred on the in-person, material sharing of a particular consumer product: food. Members enact caring relations through the provision and sharing of time, space and (edible) substance. The development of the HowToBuyWiki platform depends on activities and decisions undertaken by the organization's six active members, and the interpersonal networks between them. As we discuss in this chapter, the centrality of food in HowToBuyWiki's meetings – as a sensorially-experienced material substance that is commensally incorporated into bodies – contrasts with, and accentuates, the non-sensorial, label-based format in which the organization frames food products on its wiki-platform. In this way, HowToBuyWiki is a case study that illuminates multiple forms of food-related care which are enacted every day and which intersect in the organization itself. In looking more closely at these forms of care, we ask: how does HowToBuyWiki construct the care relations that characterize its project? And how does it frame food products, and the roles thereof, in cultivating and maintaining care relations?

Making Chocolate on a Wiki-Platform

Central to HowToBuyWiki's online platform are comparative tables, which juxtapose various brands and models of similar products (e.g. mobile telephones, e-bikes) according to a list of applicable product attributes (e.g. weight, speed). The only food product currently featured in the comparative tables is chocolate – and, more specifically, fair trade chocolate.[4] A close reading of the table – in both design and discourse – reveals that, as constructed by HowToBuyWiki, chocolate

---

4   We examine HowToBuyWiki's discursive construction of chocolate as an example of how the organization frames food products and 'conscious consumption' more generally; however, it is important to note that HowToBuyWiki's focus on fair trade chocolate products is not coincidental. Fair trade articulates concerns with labour- and sustainability-related issues, such as those connected with cocoa farming, that are central to HowToBuyWiki's vision of *the good*. And, having integrated successfully into mainstream market practices, fair trade labels also index everyday ethical consumption (cf. Low and Davenport 2005).

is a product like any other. Structured like the tables for all other products on the wiki-platform, the chocolate table presents users with factual, often quantifiable, information about the products it features – which, it should be noted, are commercial and mass-produced. In essence, the table provides a summary of the information already available on the products' wrappers. First to be featured is the brand name; then, the table names the product's flavour (milk, dark, or hazelnut), lists ingredients and allergens, and states the product's weight, the number of chocolate pieces in each packet, the percentage of fat content, the product's organic label (if known), the percentage of cocoa content, and the product's country of origin. The table also includes an image for each of the products. Notably, just as the table restricts the 'flavour' attribute to the factual triad of milk, dark, or hazelnut, it limits the images of the products themselves to their wrappers alone. Thus, the table includes no sensory information on the chocolate products themselves – neither visual nor descriptive; seemingly biased, experience-based details about texture, aroma, and finer distinctions of flavour are omitted in favour of information that quantifies and labels the (essentially hidden) materiality of the chocolate products featured. Chocolate, then, becomes quite literally enveloped in its brand. In the rest of the chapter, as we explore the ways in which HowToBuyWiki's members frame their project and the care relations it entails, we will return to the example of chocolate to examine how these discourses become embodied (or not) in the wiki-platform's representation of this food product.

Organizing Around 'Conscious Consumption'

HowToBuyWiki was founded in 2006 by a self-described 'group of friends' – a term that was repeated in each of the interviews. While membership has fluctuated somewhat over the years, the organization continues to be maintained by the three core founding members alongside three members who joined in 2007, 2008, and 2011, through friendship and familial networks. HowToBuyWiki, as a founding member explained, is based on a 'civil society' concept, with emphasis on independence from other organizations and interests. The group has been managing its project as a registered charitable organization, a status which, as a founding member explained, protects the members from liability for the content users post on the platform.

At the heart of HowToBuyWiki is the establishment of an open-source Internet-based platform that promotes, in the members' words, product transparency. Product transparency, as constructed on the HowToBuyWiki platform, involves providing evidence-based information on various (user-selected) attributes of products, and the placement of similar products in direct comparison, such that users can compare attributes within different groups of product, or 'product categories'. HowToBuyWiki structures knowledge on products in table format: in each product category, various brands and models of similar products (e.g. mobile telephones, e-bikes) (rows) are tabulated against a list of applicable product attributes (e.g. weight, speed, ingredients, fuel efficiency) (columns). In principle, products and attributes are limited only by user preference; insofar as attributes are meant to reflect user priorities, product data must be entered by users – or, as the members call them, 'editors' – and comparisons can be tailored to user needs. The HowToBuyWiki website is open to everyone and currently has approximately 4,000 visitors per month, on average; however, if a reader wishes to become an editor, s/he must learn how to contribute to the HowToBuyWiki database – a process which requires some time and effort. This investment of time and effort is, however, the only hurdle to becoming an editor; HowToBuyWiki's members do not employ a vetting process, and some members said they expect that product manufacturers will also join the wiki-platform as editors.

Underlying HowToBuyWiki's vision of product transparency is the members' self-identification as 'conscious consumers'. While the members' individual understandings of 'conscious consumption' have not been incorporated definitively into HowToBuyWiki's mission statement, they share an implicit commonality:

> In the group ... there is some kind of common sense about, about conscious consuming. (...) in the meetings, we haven't had so much discussions actually about this, because it's more like implicit that we, we have a similar vision (E)

However unarticulated, 'conscious consumption', as constructed on the HowToBuyWiki platform, is both informed and conscientious, and is the main focus of care. Premised on the assumption that lack of transparency – lack of comparative knowledge or information about products – is what impedes consumer action, HowToBuyWiki engages in a data-centric form of consciousness-raising as a means to careful consumption. Although HowToBuyWiki focuses on the structuring and sharing of product information, rather than on product rating or recommendations, the members envision the platform as facilitating particular types of consumer action. In particular, the site was established as a response to companies and producers, implicitly understood as entities which cannot be trusted to act in a caring way towards their employees, consumers or the environment. For instance, upon founding the platform, the group set out to create product categories to exemplify how HowToBuyWiki might be used. They chose to compare mobile telephones, where the main focus was radiation values and their health impacts, and cars, where the main focus was carbon emissions. As one member explained, the two foci were chosen as they related to 'ecological impact', and represented categories of information not easily searchable. Thus, while the members did not rate mobile telephones or cars by 'ecological impact', they placed the information they provided, without (explicit) judgment, as a key element of 'conscious consumption'. Likewise, the wiki-platform's chocolate category features attributes through which the members implicitly frame 'conscious consumption'. The chocolate products the table compares are all labelled fair trade – indeed, the table is named 'Fair trade chocolate in comparison' – and the absence of other chocolate products suggests an implicit linking of 'conscious consumer' identities and fair trade labels (cf. Barnett et al. 2005). However, through including 'organic labels' and 'country of origin' among the attributes, the members highlight that, in addition to fair trade, conscious consumers should be aware of other product features that have ethical (and, in this case, ecological) bearing.

The form of care that HowToBuyWiki promotes, then, positions 'conscious consumption' at its core. As an organization, HowToBuyWiki members care for their (imagined) user public through facilitating heretofore difficult-to-realize 'conscious consumption', and thereby enabling users to become informed, and then (potentially) take action by changing their purchasing habits. At the same time, HowToBuyWiki constructs 'conscious consumption' as *careful* consumer action. That is, being careful in time and global space – to protect health, wellbeing and the environment in the present and for the future. In promoting transparency, the group also seeks to cultivate careful consumers, ones who make informed and conscientious decisions that consider the placement of each product, and purchasing decision thereof, within a network of environmental and other ethical relations. Fuelled by comparative information, consumer decisions, as facilitated through the HowToBuyWiki platform, are never neutral: they are always-already imbued with questions of care.

The group members' discourses of 'conscious consumption' materialized in their choices of interview venues. When we contacted the members to arrange interviews, we suggested meeting in any space of their choice. Three of the members chose to meet in urban spaces that underlined a particular vision of 'conscious consumption'. In the venue chosen by member F, progressive politics and 'conscious consumption' are explicitly linked. The venue – a restaurant located in a multifunctional building that includes meeting rooms, offices, a public sauna, a pool, and a performance space – has a long history as a public meeting space, having been founded and used by the local workers' movement, the women's movement, and other social reformers. Today, the restaurant offers a variety of 'traditional' dishes prepared with locally-sourced, seasonally available ingredients. Another interview took place in a café/bar located in a converted office block in the industrial part of town which is now visibly gentrified. Similarly to the restaurant described above, this is a multifunctional space that houses a book/magazine shop and a performance stage. The third café we visited had a similar gentrified industrial look, with a menu focusing on fresh foods and a variety of coffee concoctions. A local contact described the interview venues as frequented by young professionals with an apparent artistic or intellectual bent, who 'consciously consume' foods and spaces.

Caring about 'The Good'

HowToBuyWiki members endorse a number of values central to their vision of 'conscious consumption' – values that can be described under the headings of fairness and sustainability. When we asked HowToBuyWiki's members which issues mattered most to them individually, responses gravitated to the same categories: fair trade, ethical labour practices, durability and reliability, and ecological impact. These issues, as one member explained, are all linked through the common thread of seeking *the good*:

> [What matters is] that these are the products which are produced in a good way. And 'good' means for me good for the nature, good for the people who make them. (D)

Like ideas of 'nature' (Castree 1995), ideas of *the good* are neither self-evident nor universal. As Williams (1995) argues in his article on diverging discourses of the 'public good' in opposing social movements, while rhetorics of *the good* appeal to an imagined consensus, they actually speak to group identities and actions. In their interviews, HowToBuyWiki's members did not discuss or debate what constitutes good products; their notions of goodness had already been established, and, as demonstrated in an earlier quote, made implicit, even tacit. And these notions of goodness were rooted in a mapping of careful global citizenship. A good product was one that was deemed to have positive impact within the broad ecology of production and consumption, with certain entities (labourers and the environment) being primary beneficiaries, and others (government, industry, retailers) placed lower on the hierarchy. To consume consciously, then, is to adhere to a vision of *the good* whereby the consumer, as a critical entity, cares for disadvantaged entities in the market economy. On the wiki-platform, this framing is apparent in HowToBuyWiki's exclusion of all non-fair trade chocolate products from its comparative table, and in its emphasis on 'organic labels' and 'country of origin' – indicators of labour- and sustainability-related concerns.

Although HowToBuyWiki's members all said they are committed to 'conscious consumption', they also explained that their personal convictions do not guide the construction of the wiki platform. Rather than place issues of sustainability and justice as the core of their project, they said, the group situates public participation as its main value. This focus on public participation is closely linked to the very founding of HowToBuyWiki, a process that started beyond the market context; indeed, the 'origin myth' of HowToBuyWiki, as one of the founders related it, is located in a public library. It was there, during a city planning project, that the three founding members converged, witnessing first-hand the involvement of the public (in this case, city residents) in making a decision about a project that would affect them all:

> [this city planning project] is surely something which brought us the idea how important – it has nothing to do with consumption, but – it was about participation and um, expressing an opinion, you know (...) we thought it would be also, if we offered the platform, there would be enough consumers who would be motivated enough to share their knowledge, motivated by the idea that they can help someone take a consumption decision which is well, um, argued. (C)

What initially inspired the founding members, then, was the idea of involving the public (implicitly positioned as having less power, awareness, and potential influence than the 'conscious consumer') in larger-scale decision-making. This idea has remained central to the way HowToBuyWiki views itself and the product – the platform – it provides to consumers. Moving away from (direct) focus on the causes nearest to the members, HowToBuyWiki is intended to elevate public participation above the top-down promotion of particular issues. This conceptualization of care notably differs from policy and NGO configurations: HowToBuyWiki 'offer[s]' a space where people can 'share', argue, offer advice, and make their voices heard (within a defined and administrated space) – as opposed to creating a site that provides users with ready-made recommendations to incorporate and enact. As described in the above quote, HowToBuyWiki's construction of public participation is based on an assumption of altruism; just as the group 'offer[s]' the platform to the unseen public, the users, according to member C, are expected to feel 'motivated' to 'help' other, equally unseen, consumers. The group, then, entangles actions and assumptions of care as the basic foundation of its wiki-platform, with the project premised both on enactments of 'conscious consumption', and on the imagining of users as people who care.

Framing Shared Values, Caring Leaders and (Imagined) Careful Users

The members of HowToBuyWiki, while committed to constructing a participatory platform, continue to be committed to consumption decisions that foster *the good*. This dual commitment is not without conflict, and the relative salience of each value – public participation and *the good* – has shifted over time. In the words of one of the founders:

> I think in the beginning it was more, there was a stronger normative touch to it. That we thought this should be a site – where we can see which products are good and we promote, you know, like, promoting a sustainable way of doing consumption, and I think we are moving slightly away from that. That I think we are still normative of course, but more on a second level. That we say we want transparency and not evaluation of products, you know? (A)

As this member implied, HowToBuyWiki's evolution from the evaluation of products to (apparently) neutral transparency – now the core of the project – is aligned with the members' original emphasis on public participation as the project's leading value. Thus, rather than promoting 'normative' constructs of sustainability and justice, HowToBuyWiki now promotes an open platform which aims to foreground the users' own preferences and voices, rather than those of the organization's members.

Yet, while HowToBuyWiki members cite the platform's openness as central to its ethos (and even its *raison d'être*), this openness also leads to difficulty in imagining how HowToBuyWiki might be administrated. In the interviews, we posed a hypothetical scenario to the members: What would happen if two users posted conflicting information about the same product? Would there be room for two narratives, for conflict? How would you decide which information would appear on the site? Their answers highlighted the ambiguity inherent in this situation.

> I can imagine that we can open a discussion forum in order to ask if the broader, the wider community, what their opinion is. Umm, I don't know. (…) But what we don't want is that we decide about what should stay on the platform. We don't want it, we really want to, just to give it, this platform, to our, to our editors. (…) my ideal would be that they should decide. (C)

> Do we, do we have the right to um, to edit some of the information which is put up by other people? Because then it becomes crucial. But because in the beginning it was really thought of as a participatory project, and everybody has the right to upload anything according to their, to the guidelines of the project. (E)

This scenario, while hypothetical, revealed central definitional concerns for HowToBuyWiki's members. In the interviews, each of the members engaged deeply with this question, speaking out an internal debate without attempting to polish uncertainties into clear-cut responses. Centering the debate in the question of editing, the members discursively negotiated their practical role as wiki-platform administrators with their vision of creating an open, community-led platform. Thus, although HowToBuyWiki's members could conceivably judge between reliable and unreliable information, they expressed the concern that to endorse certain 'truths' on the platform would amount to backtracking on their ethos. As member E argued, HowToBuyWiki members did not 'have the right' to act as arbitrators of truth. Rather, the platform, suggested member C, belonged to HowToBuyWiki's members only insofar as it was theirs to *give away*. In this instance, caring for users did not mean guaranteeing the accuracy of information on the platform, but rather maintaining the integrity of the vision that underlay it.

While cast as central to HowToBuyWiki's ethos, the openness of the platform also has the potential to jeopardize the 'conscious consumption' goals of HowToBuyWiki's members – who, after all, aim to foster consumption decisions that facilitate *the good*. When structuring product categories, users might not share the priorities that HowToBuyWiki's members endorse, and might privilege certain attributes (e.g. price) over others (e.g. carbon footprint) in ways that do not align with HowToBuyWiki's aims. However, in practice, as the members explain, their open platform continues to facilitate 'normative' discourses – in ways that perhaps do not undermine the project's ethos, but do make it more ambivalent:

> [W]e tried to ask, if we realize the potential consumers – editors, sorry – the potential editors. They have other needs. Um, and important criteria to share

their knowledge. Maybe we can – leave it open. We can leave it open. Um, but for us, these are still aspects we focus on, and when you go to the webpage this is something which you can actually … it becomes visible when you visit there that these are the issues which are important for us. (C)

As member C pointed out, while HowToBuyWiki aims to provide an inclusive platform that would meet the diverse needs of users, the platform, in effect, directs users toward a particular form of engagement. Having created pages for product categories as examples of how the platform might be used, the members of HowToBuyWiki structured tables of product attributes that privilege the group's own priorities. As such, they not only made their own priorities visible, but also created a template – however unintentionally – that could focus future users/ editors on certain product attributes over others. As the example of the chocolate table demonstrates, while the members avoid the inclusion of product attributes that might be biased by individual experience (e.g. texture, aroma), their choice to include 'fair trade labels', 'organic labels', and 'country of origin', and exclude price-related information, frames which attributes are the expected foci. Yet this latent 'normativity', as one founding member explained, is not necessarily opposed to the project's ethos of openness:

But we want to make it easy so that they can also take into consideration this specific value which is very much being suppressed by the communication of the company. (A)

Although fostering an open platform may be HowToBuyWiki's form of caring for the user public, this openness is meant, ultimately, to facilitate the project's main aim – promoting product transparency. Users are expected to use the platform in particular ways: to employ its openness to demand hidden or difficult-to-obtain information, to imagine which heretofore ignored product attributes should be brought into the forefront, to contest information and demand evidence. As HowToBuyWiki's members envision them, the users, then, are meant to use the platform's openness *with* and *for* care, of themselves, others, the environment, and their health. The platform is not merely a *tabula rasa* the users are 'given' (to use member C's earlier term); rather, being cared for through an open forum, they are expected to reciprocate with careful, altruistic, and goodness-driven action.

Caring as/for Consumers

In developing an open, community-based wiki platform, HowToBuyWiki's members both assume and relinquish leadership of their project: they are social entrepreneurs who aim to 'give' their project to users, who envision their project's agenda being set by the public. At the same time, they do not imagine themselves as being clearly separate from the public to whom they reach out. As mentioned earlier, HowToBuyWiki endorses a 'civil society' concept, and members emphasize their organization's independence from all other bodies – governmental, commercial, and even third-sector. As such, while at times drawing distinctions between 'members' and 'users' (as seen in the previous section), HowToBuyWiki's members also discursively identify as consumers – and, specifically, as part of the platform's user public. For example, when explaining why s/he found it valuable to be involved in HowToBuyWiki, member B said,

> [HowToBuyWiki] would definitely make also my life easier if it would exist and would function. Um, because I'm also consuming products every day. And I often find it difficult to find free and comparable information which is, um, useful to me. (B)

While, in this instance, member B clearly identified as a consumer who might benefit from HowToBuyWiki, aligning oneself with the user public was also achieved through less direct discourses. When we asked member D, 'What do you know currently about the people who are contributing to the site?', s/he replied:

> I know that there are not only consumers, but also producers who write on the site. (...) we thought that it's not bad, because they are – we actually give them like the structure where they have to fill in the information. It means that even though it's the producer's side, but the consumer side gives ... the contents which we want to know. And most of that, these are not the contents that they always want to share with us. (D)

In this excerpt, member D seamlessly merged 'we' as HowToBuyWiki members and 'we' as consumers. This discursive merging was telling: while HowToBuyWiki aims to facilitate user-generated (as opposed to member-generated) priorities and structuring of knowledge, member D aligned HowToBuyWiki's interests with those of the user public. The 'us' versus 'them' dynamic that appeared in member D's response invoked members and users versus producers, firmly situating the project in consumer-based origins and agendas.

While HowToBuyWiki's members discursively position themselves as consumers, they also distinguish themselves from the public(s) for whom they care – by virtue of responsibility, not expertise. As self-described 'conscious consumers', the members identify themselves as possessing awareness and conscientiousness that align them with a particular segment of the public. By itself, this identification does not set the members apart from (potential) users. When we asked the members to describe how they imagined the wiki-platform's users, each member said that the users of the site are most likely to be people who care about making informed consumption decisions, have awareness of particular consumption issues, and are actively searching for information about consumer products. The members' imaginings of these users' needs are actualized, discursively, in the wiki-platform's comparative tables. For example, the chocolate table features information on sustainability- and labour-related attributes, alongside information on allergens, underscoring that while the members conceptualize 'conscious consumption' as ethical consumption, they also imagine that some users are drawn to their site for other information needs. Indeed, the organization's meeting notes specifically state that the project's target population could be consumers with diabetes, or consumers who follow a kosher diet (Minutes of meeting, 01/02/2008).

The imagined users largely resemble the members' own 'conscious consumer' profiles. However, what sets HowToBuyWiki's members apart from other 'conscious consumers' is the sense of bearing a special social responsibility. As seen in previous sections, members spoke of 'offering' the wiki platform to the public, of 'giving' it away – altruistic acts of fostering the public good. Another recurrent discourse was that of being involved in HowToBuyWiki despite lacking resources and, especially, time. In the interviews, each participant mentioned that all members had full-time jobs and busy lives, and that HowToBuyWiki was a 'spare-time' project, even a 'hobby'. This discourse was invoked, mostly, to explain the slow progress of the site; however, it was also used to underscore the importance that members ascribed to their project, and the pride with which they engaged in it.

> [E]very one of us is very, very busy and we do it just by, because, as I said, because we're doing something which is good (laughs), which would have a good impact and which consumers can really work and benefit from. (C)

Involvement in the project, then, is not merely a pleasurable challenge, or an exercise in activism; it is imbued with a sense of social responsibility. Several members said they had no stake in the success of HowToBuyWiki as individuals, and that they would be glad if another organization developed a similar platform with greater success. Yet, they explained that they continued to be involved in the project given its (apparent) uniqueness in the consumer activist landscape. This uniqueness of the platform – its formulation as caring for consumers through openness, public participation, and transparency – was bound with a sense that the members themselves bore special responsibility for the realization of the project. As one founding member said, albeit with a humourous tone, when talking about the beginnings of the organization: 'And yeah ... then we thought we (laughs) if not we, who else would do something about food transparency?'

'Conscious consumption' and social responsibility, however, did not translate into (claims of) expertise. Indeed, throughout the interviews, HowToBuyWiki's members discursively set themselves apart from those they considered 'professional' experts in the consumer protection arena. Such discourses of 'us' (lay) and 'them' (experts) were most pronounced when the members discussed plans for installing an Advisory Board. The Advisory Board, which has since been convened, now includes advisors who represent academic, political, and social entrepreneurship angles on consumer protection. At the time of the interviews, when the Advisory Board was still being discussed, we asked the members about plans for convening the Board.

> [We'd like to] install the Advisory Board, also to um, first of all, to get some feedback on the project and of people who deal with consumer protection and um, know, know what's going on in that field, because that's not our profession. We are doing this in our, as I said, in our spare time, as a kind of a hobby. (B)

> [S]o we actually wanted to have this professional background on which we could um, we can um, lean on and on the other side it's good for us, or for the project, it's good to have the Advisory Board with names on it which are known (…) as professionals. Knowing that what they say that's, that's [authoritative] in some communities (…) especially in scientific communities. (D)

The line that member B drew between HowToBuyWiki's members and the potential advisors was clear: the former are lay activists who, without the 'professional' expertise of the latter, have neither the time nor the experience to move the project forward. For member D, however, the boundary was less clearly defined. According to member D, while the Advisory Board would provide 'professional' expertise on which HowToBuyWiki can rely and build its future activities, the inclusion of known experts as advisors to the project would also be strategic, providing the project with recognition, legitimacy, and an authoritative tone it would not otherwise achieve. Member D's account of the Advisory Board points to an underlying question of impact. Although the project places public participation, and the leveling of authority, as its defining characteristic – the uniqueness that justifies its existence – the reality of the project, in which members have struggled for years to recruit users/editors, suggests that the wiki-platform has yet to gain momentum, or even a stable user base. Turning to a more 'traditional' model of expertise, based in individuals of renown, rather than in a faceless user community, HowToBuyWiki's members both concede the need for authoritative endorsement, and strategically solidify their self-identification as non-experts; it is their lay status, they suggest, not the actual merit of the project, which has impeded the platform's success with potential users. With the convening of the Advisory Board, the division of labour becomes clearer: the Board members are there to provide legitimacy and expert support, but the organization's members are those who provide care, and mobilize both experts and companies to care, too.

Facilitating or Empowering Careful Action?

In keeping with the participatory ethos of their project, HowToBuyWiki's members cast themselves as responsible for the development and maintenance of an online platform – not for the provision of information. Their role, they argue, is to enable users to 'organiz[e] information', structure knowledge, and provide product data meaningful to them:

> [I]t's critical. It is not us who can make it move forward, I mean publish the content. It's not the idea that we do the content. We just want to, to offer the platform, but it is the editors and the consumers who should fill it with content. (C)

> The information, we won't provide it. It has to be either the producers or retailers or the consumers. But we want to put in place a structure which allows for a different way of organizing information. Making it accessible, distributing information. (A)

Although HowToBuyWiki's members have provided content for certain product categories, to exemplify how the platform might be used, they view their stepping back from content-provision as crucial to the project's aim and future. Elsewhere in member A's interview, s/he explained that HowToBuyWiki members can contribute information, but only as individual consumers, not under the aegis of their organization. However, as evident in member C's quote, while HowToBuyWiki's members may still (strategically) identify as consumers, they simultaneously draw a line between themselves and their user public. Thus, when it comes to engaging with the wiki-platform, boundaries between members and users become more apparent, with members providing infrastructure, while users populate the site.

As described by members, then, HowToBuyWiki's main role is *facilitation*, and the form of care that members provide to consumers is one of enabling the structuring and sharing of information as the latter see fit. Yet, as member A implied in the excerpt above, the organization's focus on facilitating user engagement is not entirely neutral. In member A's construction of user engagement, the wiki-platform would provide space for dialogue – dialogue, which, notably, would occur not just between consumers, but also between consumers, retailers, and producers. Indeed, the wiki community member A envisions not only shares information, but also demands it:

> [Producers] in HowToBuyWiki now have to enter a dialogue, and have to provide this and structure this information in dialogue with other producers and in dialogue with the consumers. Yeah I think this is a fundamental change, I think this is very, very, different from advertisement. (…) And the idea is to say … the consumers also have a certain power, by consuming or not consuming, but they need to organize their interests and discourses which are important to them in a certain way that maybe yeah, as I said, forces the producers to enter a dialogue with them. (A)

Member A, then, cast HowToBuyWiki as poised to create a new power dynamic. According to member A, through providing consumers with an open, participatory wiki-platform, HowToBuyWiki would foreground consumers' voices and needs, and thereby highlight the power that consumers hold. The dialogue s/he imagined – a dialogue based on the categorizing and structuring of product information – would therefore overturn the extant vectors of the market. In alluding to advertising, member A underscored the (perceived) unidirectionality of communication between producers and consumers, and the suggested subversiveness of the wiki-platform, where consumers, no longer mere recipients of (potentially manipulative) messaging, would talk back. HowToBuyWiki, then, could empower consumers: to acknowledge and affirm their economic importance, make demands of producers, and take informed – 'conscious' – action. In this conceptualization of HowToBuyWiki, the organization would be a driving force for consumer empowerment through shifting dynamics of agency and power. Such an overtly politicized stance, and the neoliberal visions of responsibilized consumers to which it alludes, might seem to be at odds with the form of care espoused by HowToBuyWiki's members, one which emphasizes community and facilitation. Yet, as member A argued explicitly, and as other members suggested more implicitly, HowToBuyWiki members view 'conscious consumption' as one which, of necessity, would alter the landscape of the market. Careful consumers, they posit, will establish not only the value of disadvantaged entities (labourers, the environment), but also their own position at the crux of the market economy.

Forming a Nexus of Care Relations

The forms of care that HowToBuyWiki's members described – the careful actions enacted through the wiki-platform – are not the only careful actions that underlie HowToBuyWiki. Practices such as sharing time, food, and social activities have been central to the making and sustaining of HowToBuyWiki from its inception, and members all describe their involvement in the project and the attendant meetings as a way of strengthening their friendships. As other researchers have emphasized, friendship ties are important in maintaining SCMOs (Forno and Graziano 2014; Grasseni 2013; Parigi and Gong 2014). However, in the case of HowToBuyWiki, the organization itself can be seen as a platform for cultivating attentiveness to, and care relations with, one's friends.

When asked about how they keep in contact, members explained that day-to-day contact was maintained through email, telephone, and Skype, but that face-to-face meetings were much more important. Records of care practices feature centrally in the organization's otherwise brief agendas and meeting minutes. The first board meeting was accompanied by 'a glass of champagne and bacon pancakes' (Founding meeting agenda, 08/02/2006). While matters of taste and preference are omitted in the group's online characterization of chocolate, the members attend to personal tastes and preferences in their meeting minutes. To-do lists for each member prior to a weekend workshop included specific project-related tasks, as well as the light-hearted reminder to '[r]eport any special requests for pizza toppings and breakfast supplies to [member A]' (Workshop schedule, 10/08/2013).

The project is also an initiative through which members' friends and families can practise caring relations. These relations are expressed through the provision of money, encouragement and in-kind support. Initial plans for HowToBuyWiki were validated by experts as well as friends and family: 'University friends – find the idea very good' (Minutes of meeting, 04/04/2008); this support from friends is noted in the minutes in a list which also includes records of positive responses from academic experts and other supporting information. Meetings are held at the homes of members or their families. At an early stage of the project, the father of one of the members wanted to donate money to support the project (Minutes of meeting, 04/03/2008). This suggestion is echoed in later records; a means for formally accepting donations was devised by the group and several 'generous donations' were received, the most recent in 2013 (Minutes of AGM, 10/08/2013). Members also care for each other through support and encouragement, and by celebrating small successes: 'This report was greeted with raging applause', read AGM minutes, 'the continuation of the project was unanimously supported' (Minutes of AGM, 19/02/2011). In this way, HowToBuyWiki is not simply an internet platform, but an entity which catalyzes and facilitates a network of care between and around its members.

Discussion: Matters of Care

In the scheme of caring relations constructed by HowToBuyWiki's members, the members themselves care for consumers (through developing and maintaining the wiki-platform), while the (cared-for) consumers, in turn, are expected to care for other consumers (through sharing knowledge), as well as for labourers, the environment, and their own wellbeing (through making 'conscious consumption' decisions). Yet, although this directionality of care may seem to be clear-cut, the nature of HowToBuyWiki's caring action, as conceptualized by the organization's members, is imbued with ambiguities. Throughout the interviews, the members spoke alternately of enabling and empowering users, informing and educating the public, and locating expertise in individuals and in communities. While these pairings do not constitute polar contradictions, they do highlight the multiform nature of care in which HowToBuyWiki's members engage. Caring for consumers, as the members spoke of it, could equally be enacted through providing users with a platform that promotes certain 'conscious consumption' values, and through offering users an open platform, free of judgement and evaluation. Although HowToBuyWiki has shifted toward the latter form of care, in their accounts of their own identities, roles, and goals *vis-à-vis* the project, the members indicated that the realities of the organization's acts of caring borrow from both forms, and are situated (albeit sometimes tensely) in a terrain of fruitful ambiguity.

Central to HowToBuyWiki's project is the act of *mobilizing for care*. In the interviews, the members mapped a network of care, one in which their organization holds a critical position. Comprised of key entities placed along a hierarchy of authority to care, this network relies on the different actions that, according to HowToBuyWiki's members, each entity is expected to take. The chain of caring action, as conceptualized by the members, is set in motion by HowToBuyWiki, which mobilizes expert support (the Advisory Board) and facilitates 'conscious consumers'' caring actions. In the reaction (anticipated) to follow, 'conscious consumers' (editors and users) mobilize the general public (who then join the ranks of 'conscious consumption'), and put pressure on producers (for product transparency); experts (the Advisory Board) inform and legitimize HowToBuyWiki, thus further strengthening the organization's empowerment of 'conscious consumers'; and producers respond to consumer pressure by contributing information to HowToBuyWiki. However, absent from HowToBuyWiki's network are all governmental institutions. While some members mentioned certain policy-makers in their interviews, they did so in the context of discussions about the Advisory Board, discussions which, notably, evoked political figures as opinion-leaders, rather than as policy-makers. HowToBuyWiki's network of care, then, is market-driven, with consumption as the currency of influence. In this network, consumers are politically empowered through realizing, and acting on, their purchasing power: a neoliberal vision that casts individual users as rational decision-makers, responsible for their own choices, atomized though (paradoxically) linked as an online community. HowToBuyWiki's members thus configure caring for consumers as, essentially, enabling them to practise informed self-care.

While HowToBuyWiki was established for the purposes of caring for and about others – consumers, exploited workers, or future populations who may face problems resulting from environmental change – and while members construct a complex network of care, in which their organization is centrally positioned, a different form of caring is identifiable in the day-to-day practices of the group. The members who launched the project were friends who shared common but unstated values. They began to discuss how they might be able to have an impact on the world with respect to these values, and HowToBuyWiki grew out of these discussions. While HowToBuyWiki has not managed to develop a stable community of users and editors, it has achieved its implicit project – that of members caring for their friendship group. The sort of everyday, interpersonal care described by Jespersen et al. (2014) is evident in the way that group members collaborate. The group functions well because members listen to each other and respond to one another's needs; emotional and personal relationships are entangled amongst group members, and the project serves as a way for them to see each other regularly. The importance of interpersonal care for the success of HowToBuyWiki, and vice-versa, is evident from the meeting minutes and workshop programmes in which food, social dinners, drinks and dancing are frequently planned alongside workshopping the web interface and writing funding proposals.

Where is food in the forms of care relations discussed here? On the one hand, on the HowToBuyWiki platform, food is just one product among many others: its ingredients and modes of production are, at least structurally, of equal weight to those of, for example, a deodorant. On the other hand, in HowToBuyWiki's meetings, food is a substance whose production and consumption are shared and carefully noted in meeting minutes. Here, food is central not only to interpersonal care relations, but also to the building and maintenance of the organization. While the platform is populated with images of packaging, lists of ingredients, and eco-labels, the organization's meeting minutes are populated with foods which, for HowToBuyWiki members, are fresh, seasonal, local, pleasurable, and not necessarily imbued with variable attributes. Focusing on care therefore points to one significant difference between food as experienced and food as commoditized (or between 'food' and 'food products'), and raises questions about the extent to which processes of globalization and technological development might reconfigure caring through food.

Although the project's success may be secondary to the group's interpersonal acts of care, the project itself continues to be essential to their maintenance: through the process of establishing, maintaining, and editing the HowToBuyWiki platform, the members' acts of caring for one another (and for the wider public) are now bound with the object of care – the platform itself. '[T]ransforming things into matters of care', argues Puig de la Bellacasa, 'is a way of relating to them, of inevitably becoming affected by them, and of modifying their potential to affect others' (2011: 99). For HowToBuyWiki's members, the platform becomes imbued not only with the values of 'conscious consumption' that underpin the project, but also with the affective social relationships this project has helped develop and maintain over time. A non-human object of care, then, can define its human carer; or, as Heuts and Mol argue in their study of 'good tomatoes' and the experts who care for and about them: 'the values targeted, the objects being valued and valuing subjects come to gradually co-constitute each other' (2013: 141).

The example of HowToBuyWiki illustrates the complexity and multidirectionality of care. The initiative permeates the virtual and the non-virtual, and collapses the boundary between 'caring' and 'cared-for'. HowToBuyWiki's project is premised on a chain of care relations which, though not always directly reciprocal, implicate members and users in giving and receiving care: members care for users through providing the wiki-platform, while users care for HowToBuyWiki by accepting this action of care and contributing to the platform, thereby also caring for one another through sharing information. In the organization itself, the members cultivate their care relations through regular meetings in which they attend to one another, organizing weekends away, engaging in small collaborations in pairs, sharing food, encouraging each other's efforts, and celebrating small successes. With no clear-cut dichotomy between giver and recipient, HowToBuyWiki exemplifies how care is not only an outcome-orientated process of improvement (cf. Heuts and Mol 2013), but is also a practice of sharing time and attention, which is essential for creating and maintaining a community.

Acknowledgements

This chapter is based on research funded by the Oxford Martin School's Programme for the Future of Food. We would like to thank our research project's Principal Investigator, Professor Stanley Ulijaszek, and Co-Principal Investigators Dr. Catherine Dolan and Dr. Javier Lezaun. We would also like to thank the members of HowToBuyWiki for generously sharing their experiences and official documents with us.

References

Balsiger, P. 2013. *Embedding 'Political Consumerism': A Conceptual Critique.* EUI Working Paper MWP 2013/08. San Domenico di Fiesole: European University Institute.

Barnes, M. 2012. *Care in Everyday Life: An Ethic of Care in Practice.* Bristol: Policy Press.

Barnett, C., Cloke, P., Clarke, N. and Malpass, A. 2005. Consuming ethics: Articulating the subjects and spaces of ethical consumption. *Antipode*, 37(1), 23-45.

Castree, N. 1995. The nature of produced nature: Materiality and knowledge production in Marxism. *Antipode*, 27(1), 12-48.

Forno, F. and Graziano, P.R. 2014. Sustainable community movement organisations. *Journal of Consumer Culture*, 14(2), 139-57.

Gilligan, C. 1982. *In a Different Voice.* Cambridge MA: Harvard University Press.

Grasseni, C. 2013. *Beyond Alternative Food Networks: Italy's Solidarity Purchase Groups.* London: Berg/Bloomsbury Academic.

Heuts, F. and Mol, A. 2013. What is a good tomato? A case of valuing in practice. *Valuation Studies*, 1(2), 125-46.

Jespersen, A.P., Bønnelycke, J. and Eriksen, H.H. 2014. Careful science? Bodywork and care practices in randomised clinical trials. *Sociology of Health & Illness*, 36(5), 655-69.

Lacey, A. 2005. Networked communities: Social centers and activist spaces in contemporary Britain. *Space and Culture*, 8(3), 286-301.

London, A.J. and Kadane, J.B. 2003. Sham surgery and genuine standards of care: Can the two be reconciled? *The American Journal of Bioethics*, 3(4), 61-4.

Low, W. and Davenport, E. 2005. Postcards from the edge: Maintaining the 'alternative' character of fair trade. *Sustainable Development*, 13(3), 143-53.

Micheletti, M. 2003. *Political Virtue and Shopping: Individuals, Consumerism, and Collective Action.* Houndsmills, Basingstoke, New York: Palgrave Macmillan.

Mol, A., Moser, I. and Pols, J. 2010. Care: Putting practice into theory, in *Care in Practice: On Tinkering in Clinics, Homes and Farms*, edited by A. Mol, I. Moser J. and Pols, Bielefeld: Transcript Verlag, 7-26.

Parigi, P. and Gong, R. 2014. From grassroots to digital ties: A case study of a political consumerism movement. *Journal of Consumer Culture*, 14(2), 236-53.

Puig de la Bellacasa, M. 2011. Matters of care in technoscience: Assembling neglected things. *Social Studies of Science*, 41(1), 85-106.

Reavley, N.J., Morgan, A.J., Jorm, D. and Jorm, A.F. 2013. An evaluation of mental health wiki: A consumer guide to mental health information on the Internet. *Journal of Consumer Health on the Internet*, 17(1), 1-9.

Sutton, D., Naguib, N., Vournelis, L. and Dickinson, M. 2013. Food and contemporary protest movements. *Food, Culture and Society: An International Journal of Multidisciplinary Research*, 16(3), 345-66.

Thomas, C. 1993. De-constructing concepts of care. *Sociology*, 27(4), 649-69.

Tronto, J.C. 1993. *Moral Boundaries: A Political Argument for an Ethic of Care*. London: Routledge.

Williams, R.H. 1995. Constructing the public good: Social movements and cultural resources. *Social Problems*, 42(1), 124-44.

Chapter 9

Children's Engagements with Food: An Embodied Politics of Care through School Meals

Mónica Truninger and José Teixeira

Introduction

In Portugal, since the 1970s food made available in schools has played a chief role in the wider strategy of democratizing education through caring for children's wellbeing (Nunes de Almeida 2011; Stoer 1983). During this time, school meals have undergone gradual changes and innovations. These have been shaped by diverse rationalities and dynamics of power emerging from shifting processes in the organization of children's food practices. These processes include: decentralization and privatization of the management of school meal services; the implementation of new food safety regulations; the setting up of modern cooking equipment; improving the nutritional value of school menus and the food portions made available to children; changing cooking practices; and limiting the kinds of food provided in schools' coffee shops or vending machines (Truninger et al. 2013). Despite some degree of adaptation, the design of these policies has tended to favour children's engagement with school meals through their minds – to change their understandings of health and nutrition – thereby marginalizing their bodies, and the visceral effects of food intake. In this chapter we argue that these changes to the legal framework of school meals have been influenced by multiple rationalities, such as nutrition, economics, environment, social justice, and culture. These have impacted on how care is mobilized in the context of school meal practices (i.e. their regulation, management, purchasing, preparation, cooking, eating and disposal) and, hence, on the ways in which children engage with food (i.e. accepting, cooperating or rejecting the food provided).

As argued by Rummery and Fine (2012), there is a relative consensus that care is a complex process, which entails emotional and cognitive dispositions towards Others (i.e. caring *about*) and physical activities in the form of paid or unpaid labour (i.e. caring *for*). However, they call attention to the fact that care also comprises 'interpersonal relationships involving both individual and structural power dynamics' (ibid: 329). These relationships are often difficult and tense because caring is both about being attentive and responsive to someone else's needs and ensuring recognition, cooperation and social participation by care receivers.

These scholars also claim that care has become increasingly professionalized and technical, often governed by social care policies and legal frameworks that challenge ethical and emotional engagement with Others' needs (ibid: 326).

Following Wright and Harwood (2009), children's eating practices and the organization of school meals can also be framed in terms of biopedagogies. This concept is inspired by Foucault's notion of 'biopower' (1978), which frames power as being everywhere and not necessarily in the form of authority or top-down mechanisms that regulate individual bodies and eating. Thus, power also emerges from within individuals through disciplinary practices in the form of self-monitoring, surveillance, and ultimately, self-care. In this vein, biopedagogies comprise both regulatory strategies and disciplinary techniques 'that enable the governing of bodies in the name of health and life' (Wright and Harwood 2009: 8). Acting as regulatory strategies, they are shaped by 'discourses of truth' based upon multiple rationales legitimizing particular regimes of 'governmentality' (Miller and Rose 2008). That is to say that biopedagogies draw 'attention to the pedagogical practices inhering in the biopolitical (for example, public health promotion)' (Wright and Harwood 2009: 21). Acting as disciplinary techniques, biopedagogies affect subjectivities that are produced, circulated and embodied. For example, in the case of school meals, subjects work on themselves in order to discipline their bodies and food tastes.

By engaging with school meal practices, authorities and kitchen staff make use of such biopedagogies as mechanisms of subjection (regularizing) and subjectification (disciplining) to affect both entire school populations as well as individual bodies, their subjectivities and relations with food. Although biopedagogies can be seen as 'spaces of ordering', on closer examination, such modes of subjectification reveal that they can also be considered as 'spaces of resistance' that disrupt the 'homogenizing attempts of biopower' (Harwood 2009: 27).

In this chapter we show how the organization of school meals mobilizes care through the enactment of biopedagogies in their biopolitical and disciplining modes. We also show that this process can open up 'spaces of tension' or 'buffer zones' where the outcomes of rationalities and power dynamics do not necessarily manifest themselves in the form of resistance, opposition and outright rejection but instead as negotiation, continuous adjustment and 'practical tinkering' (Mol et al. 2010: 13). By contrasting both public and public-private partnership modes of food provisioning, our aim in this chapter is to look at the tensions, negotiations and adjustments that emerge from these processes. Inspired by Carolan's ideas around food 'lived experiences' (2011: 1), we think about food relationally through developing a 'subject-decentred' and generative approach to children's food practices, which takes into consideration the multiple sites of their experiences and positions them as 'becomings' rather than 'beings' (Brembeck and Johansson 2010. See also Carolan 2011). Children's practices, senses and embodiment are all key elements of our approach to their engagement with food. Rather than focusing uniquely on children's voices and relationships with food providers, we explore their food practices as interwoven with broader experiences in which bodies interact and engage with diverse socio-material arrangements.

This chapter is organized into five parts. First, we discuss the methods, the case studies and the materials collected. Then we provide a brief historical overview of the evolution of school meal policies in Portugal in order to understand what ethics of care (i.e. knowledge and understandings promoting attentive responsiveness to another's care needs) have been historically present and how they frame the organization of food practices in schools. Thirdly, we analyse how interrogating biopedagogies of school meals reveals tensions and adjustments that often emerge during the performance of non-direct forms of care, such as designing school meal policies and implementing healthy food initiatives. In the fourth section we move our focus onto children's bodies and eating practices in order to explore acceptance, negotiation and resistance strategies in which children often engage while embodying, and corporeally disrupting, school meal biopedagogies. In the final section of the chapter we make some concluding remarks about practical constraints that emerge during the organization of school meals and the benefits of perceiving an ethic of care as a process of mutual understanding wherein bodies often become entangled and negotiated things.

Methods

Our analysis is drawn from the findings of a three-year project entitled 'Between School and Family: Children's Food Knowledge and Eating Practices'[1]. This study aims to look at Portuguese school meal regulations alongside initiatives that encourage 'healthy eating', children's food knowledge and the eating practices of their families. The data were collected in four primary and four secondary schools from three different regions in Portugal: Lisbon, Vila Real and Madeira. While Lisbon is predominantly an urban and cosmopolitan region, Vila Real and Madeira combine both urban and rural areas.

A total of nine focus groups were carried out with children (five with primary school children aged between seven and nine years old, and four with secondary children aged between ten and 14 years old). We also conducted nine focus groups with parents whose children attended the eight schools selected for study. These parents were not all related, however, to children participating in the focus groups.

1   The project was supported by national science funds through the Foundation for Science and Technology (PTDC/CS-SOC/111214/2009 and PEst-OE/SADG/LA0013/2013) and the design and methods were inspired by an ESRC project hosted at Cardiff University (RES-000-23-1095). One member of the team at Cardiff University, Dr. Mara Miele, served as a consultant in our project. Dr. Miele's contribution to the conceptual thinking and research design of the project was invaluable. Notably the methods designed by Dr. Miele for the British project were replicated in this Portuguese one. The aim of this was to ensure the possibility of future comparative research.

During the discussions we explored several aspects of children's relationships with food, such as: their daily eating patterns and preferences; their participation in family food-related activities; the division of domestic food-centred labour practices, such as shopping, cooking and cleaning up; and their opinions on school meal services. During the week prior to the focus groups, children had filled in food diaries describing the meals they ate – where, at what time and with whom. Parents, in their turn, were asked to complete a brief survey for socio-demographic purposes after the focus group. Thirty-nine interviews with stakeholders (i.e. school and kitchen staff; national, regional and local authorities; nutritionists; catering firms) were conducted together with participant observation in spaces of food consumption at the schools (e.g. canteens; coffee shops; playgrounds), as well as in their surrounding areas. The analysis of several official documents (e.g. European, national and regional legislation; good practice guidelines; school meal regulations, food education programmes) was also undertaken. Interviews and focus groups were fully transcribed and analysed using NVIVO 10, together with other materials that were collected in schools such as photos and video recordings. Data were coded according to themes (and sub-themes) and the analysis took into account the relations established between these themes/nodes (e.g. links between textual and contextual information).

School Meal Biopolitics and Care in Portugal

In the years before the democratic turn in Portugal in the mid-1970s, school meals had a profoundly philanthropic and paternalistic character. Informal food provision was commonly framed as a private issue and primarily the responsibility of the mother (Nunes de Almeida 2011; Pimentel 2001). Since then, school meals have emerged as a 'public concern' alongside other social, economic, cultural and demographic changes. Welfare institutions have taken responsibility for children's eating practices by designing school menus and implementing food education programmes, applying hygiene and food safety rules, setting up canteens, regulating opening times and also by establishing standards for various procedures such as scheduling staff, contacting food suppliers and ordering goods. Although eating is usually referred to as a domestic and family-centred activity (DeVault 1991; Jackson 2009), implementing such 'vital politics' (Harwood 2009: 21) that target lifestyle improvements has led food consumption among young people to become an important subject of state surveillance and public intervention. As care became increasingly commoditized and marketized, it was no longer confined to 'household preferences' and 'has become instead an arena for social conflict, both implicit and explicit, marking out the important new social divisions and underlying tensions' (Fine 2005: 248).

Even though public concern about children's eating practices has increased more recently due to what some authors consider to be a 'moral panic' over childhood obesity (Wright and Harwood 2009), during the initial stages of the democratization of school meals in Portugal (1970s-1980s), the food provided in schools was already conceived of as a 'rational diet' that had to follow the principles of a 'balanced meal' and supply enough energy for a population mostly characterized by few economic resources and nutritionally-poor diets (Truninger et al. 2013). Thus, notions of good care in school meal practices have been commonly framed in terms of their contribution to the improvement of children's health status. This complies with a broader understanding of school meals as biopedagogies that implement and mobilize care. To recall, biopedagogies can be seen as practices through which regulatory and disciplinary mechanisms are arranged in the form of biopolitics and techniques of the self. Biopedagogies are mobilized through regulatory strategies (e.g. public policies, healthy food programmes) and self-monitoring techniques (e.g. monitoring food choices or body aesthetics, complying with values on healthy eating), to subjectify and subjugate individuals' minds and bodies to true discourses about life (Wright and Harwood 2009). They are organized by multiple forms of expert knowledge, such as biomedicine and socio-technical arrangements (e.g. school menus), and they combine diverse materials (e.g. various kinds of foods, cooking and storage equipment) and spaces, such as kitchens and canteens, coffee shops and playgrounds.

In this sense, defining standards of quality and quantity for school meals, buying and distributing food products, cooking, serving and monitoring school dinners, or negotiating the content of lunch boxes may mobilize care to govern children's eating practices and discourses, and thus, the various ways their bodies engage with food (Gibson and Dempsey 2013). The negotiations of the content of both lunch boxes and school meals are sometimes established on the basis of cooperation and mutual understanding, thus suggesting an ethic of care wherein both technical and emotional orientations towards caring *for* and *about* Others are intertwined.

During the 1990s, the number of school canteens continued to grow substantially, as did the number of children with access to school meals and other food programmes, such as free milk schemes. Yet most children still had their lunches at home. Despite their availability to almost every child, school meals were most effective at alleviating the effects of poverty and lack of access to food. Over the following years, income inequalities eased within Portuguese society and both new educational opportunities and the growth of the middle class paved the way for new habits of consumption and the development of a consumer society (Cruz 2011). Also, the management of school meals became decentralized and, in most cases, was contracted out to catering firms. Vending machines were installed in schools and a greater variety of products made available. Rather than following principles of healthy eating in schools (defined by public authorities) exclusively, the food provided was targeted at children's purchasing power and it encouraged 'consumer choice', thereby illustrating a 'marketization' of care in which children came to be envisaged as 'customers' and individually responsible for making 'healthy' choices.

As Mol points out, the logics of choice and care 'may sometimes complement each other, but more often they clash' (Mol 2008: 1). Whereas in the 1990s they seemed to complement each other rather harmoniously, with vending machines and school coffee shops offering a wide choice of foods (e.g. snacks, chocolates, fizzy drinks) alongside the single menu provided in the canteen, nowadays school children's food choices are more closely monitored in order to ensure that they follow stricter nutritional and safety guidelines. As the number of hours spent in school by primary school children has increased in tandem with their parents' working hours, the demand for formal care services for children has followed the same trend, increasing their daily consumption of school meals, especially amongst six to nine-year-olds. Additionally, concern about children's lifestyles has grown as recent studies have positioned Portugal as having some of the highest childhood overweight and obesity rates in Europe (WHO 2013). In response to this problem, healthy food initiatives (e.g. food education interventions, cooking events with chefs or healthcare professionals, BMI monitoring initiatives), food programmes (e.g. school fruit schemes) and adjustments to school meal regulations have been introduced to more rigorously control the nutritional intake of children and young people. Stricter rules for food safety and hygiene were also implemented through new European Commission food regulations in the early 2000s (e.g. HACCP)[2].

The strategic value of school meals for monitoring and improving children's health and to deal with this population's high rates of overweight/obesity has been recognized. School meals are intended to compensate for what are considered to be children's 'unhealthy' eating practices and deal with other risk factors, such as food contamination. Such aims are accomplished through rigorous procedures and rules for buying, storing and cooking; by pre-defined single option menus offering nutritionally balanced meals where the caloric value of food is made visible (see Table 9.1); by limiting the kinds of products available at school coffee shops and vending machines (e.g. crisps, chocolates, cakes); by circulating discourses on healthy lifestyles (e.g. being physically active); and through widening food choices (e.g. improving fruit, vegetable and fish intake while reducing levels of fat, sugar and salt).

---

2   Standards of hygiene and food safety were defined by Regulation (EC) n. 852/2004, Official Journal of the European Union no.139 of April 30, 2004. Parliament and European Council. Brussels.

Table 9.1   Example of two days (Monday and Tuesday) of a primary school menu in Greater Lisbon (school year 2012-13)

Day	Lunch		Calories
Monday	*Soup*	Vegetables soup	128.4
	Main dish	Grilled poultry burger with carrots and rice	528.2
	Dessert	Seasonal fruit	–
Tuesday	*Soup*	Pea soup	127.8
	Main dish	Fish pasta with salad	439.7
	Dessert	Jelly	69.8

Note: The full weekly menu was visible by the school gate.

Approaching school meal practices through the lens of 'biopower' involves taking into account the multiple 'truth' discourses about people's lives and the individuals and organizations that proclaim them. It also requires attention to population-wide strategies of intervention and modes of subjectification that are embodied by individuals across different contexts of power relations with which they interact (Miller and Rose 2008).

The mobilization of care in school meal practices is situated at multiple levels of governance, such as: policy makers' filing cabinets, municipalities, universities, school boards and catering firms, local and central kitchens, canteens, coffee shops, lunchboxes, playgrounds and schools' surrounding areas. In each of these, several actors take part in processes of decision-making that are mediated by emotional and normative orientations towards Others. In recent years, care has become increasingly mobilized through normative and regulated food practices in schools. As schools have started to be perceived as spaces of health promotion, the topic of healthy food has gained greater importance in the regulation of school meals (Carvalho 2012; Horta et al. 2013). More recently, with the moralization of children's food preferences, a particular emphasis on nutrition has been underpinned by stricter rules for food provided in schools (e.g. Decree-Law n°55/2009, and subsequent revisions through Circular n° 3/2013). Still, a different kind of approach is needed to understand how these rules are circulated and embodied in the context of micro interactions of care. That is, the particular situations where care is experienced (e.g. through self-care or bodily enactments of care by Others), in contrast to the meso and macro levels, wherein narratives of care are mediated by regulations and rearranged (e.g. through scientific, political, social and economic visions). In the following section we will draw attention to the ways in which school meal biopedagogies (in their disciplinary mode) are enacted and negotiated by policy makers' filing cabinets, school board directors, catering firms' nutritionists, serving and cooking staff.

Disciplining Children's Eating Practices in Schools: Tensions and Adjustments

In the previous section we used the concept of biopedagogies to highlight the existence of regulatory strategies impacting on school meals, such as healthy eating discourses and the regulation of school menus. However, the focus there was on the biopolitical mode of biopedagogies, which deals with the mechanisms intended to regulate and affect populations' lifestyles (the collective) rather than individuals' bodies and their subjectivities (the individual). In this section, we will look more closely at the disciplinary techniques of biopedagogies in order to explore individuals' self-awareness. This is argued to be 'mediated by their personal experiences, their own embodiment, their interactions with other ways of knowing, other truths and operations of power in relation to the knowledge produced around health, obesity and the body' (Wright 2009: 9). Although there is room for acceptance and discipline, there are also other possible tensions and outcomes to these power dynamics, such as resistance and rejection, negotiation and adjustment.

Kitchen staff are responsible for regulating children's eating practices while performing their professional duties during school time. Children, in their turn, are expected to comply with these instructions. Yet tensions emerge during these interactive processes. These can be seen within the initial stages of designing school meal regulations. As mentioned by one of the interviewees in our study – a nutritionist working in the Ministry of Education and Science – major changes in school meal regulations are dependent upon the timing of government decisions and the media agenda; they are often put under pressure by the interests of large economic and lobby groups. On one occasion, it was explained to us how policy designers had wanted to 'ban' certain kinds of foods from being available in schools, using this same terminology ('to ban') in the directives. After pressure from key economic players with interests in selling foods with excess fat, sugar or salt, such as chocolate and snacks, the policy designers were strongly encouraged to change their wording, using the milder verb 'to avoid' or the expression 'not make available' in the food recommendations for schools instead:

> We had some objectives that could not be spelt out with the exact wording we
> wanted ... namely using the term 'ban'. We wanted to ban several foods ...
> but this was not allowed by top senior officials in the ministry [of education]
> under mounting pressures from the [names a strong economic food group in the
> country] ... so the term approved was 'not make available' instead of 'to ban'
> or 'to forbid' (Interview with a representative of the Ministry of Education and
> Science, Lisbon 2011)

Although the proposals of the Ministry of Education and Science are frequently in line with expert recommendations about healthy eating, the implementation of school meal biopolitics is mediated by policy makers linked into interwoven webs of industry vested interests, media agenda setting and public expectations of 'proper' food. At times, the outcomes of these decisions contradict the advice of health professionals, which suggests that resistance may emerge even within the interstitial spaces of central government practices. In other situations, school meal guidelines do not fully comply with the recommendations of health experts, as these are not sensitive to the target population. For example, another representative of the Ministry of Education and Science recalled that once, while updating the recommended quantities of ingredients and nutrients within each meal, she had to think not only about nutritional recommendations, but also about children's taste preferences and, above all, about the effects of the current economic crisis on family budgets and consumption:

> We asked the Faculty of Sciences and Nutrition to define quantities suitable for children from pre-school to secondary school because the current ones did not take into account their age … But, reducing the quantity of meat is a difficult task nowadays … during a time of crisis, to tell a boy that instead of eating 100 grams he only needs 70 grams … it's difficult! (Interview with a representative of the Ministry of Education and Science, Lisbon, 2011)

In the end, the values suggested were slightly above the stricter nutritional recommendations, particularly of the products children liked most, because the representatives of the Ministry of Education and Science were aware of the difficulties experienced by some families, and felt that the introduction of a radical change in values, such as reducing the amount of meat and increasing the quantity of vegetables, would eventually be reflected down the line in an increase in food waste in the canteen. Without necessarily ignoring expert advice, some stakeholders are sensitive to the importance of making small adjustments to nutritional recommendations and taking account of the specificities of their target population. This example shows how caring can be adjusted at the intersection of state, taste preferences, children's bodies and broader macro-economic tendencies like the post-2008 crisis. Still, 'good care' is difficult to accomplish by means of regulatory mechanisms, as these tend to normalize values around healthy eating and children's bodies and diets.

According to school meal guidelines issued in 2009 by the Portuguese Government (Decree-Law n°55/2009 and afterwards revised by Circular n° 3/2013), following predetermined quantities for each food while preparing school meals has become mandatory. Nevertheless, when visiting school canteens and coffee shops during fieldwork, we rapidly understood how this is undermined by daily negotiations of food portions between children and serving staff. In fact, most children could ask for second helpings if they wanted (sometimes on the condition that they had eaten all of the previous serving). Nowadays, it is easy for the kitchen staff to predict the number of meals they have to prepare each day, as children must book their meals in advance through an electronic card. On the one hand, this mechanism allows catering firms to reduce their waste and economic losses, as the number of meals prepared is more accurate. On the other hand, it renders them less adaptable to last minute changes. Still, most kitchens do cater for the possibility of children wanting second helpings.

Besides the issue of food portions, ensuring the quality of the food provided in terms of its alignment with children's tastes requires overcoming various tensions. In fact, some schools have been able to maintain management of their canteen and coffee shop despite major pressures to privatize school meal services. Most of the time, this has to do with the fact that stakeholders such as school staff and even some regional authorities consider the transition to catering firms to have a negative impact on the quality of food provided:

> I've been fighting to keep the canteen under our management because I know what they are doing. If it's a company I don't know what they're doing. I said [to the dinner ladies who were asking for extra help in the kitchen]: "The day I ask for another kitchen employee, they [the Ministry of Education and Science] will shut down the canteen … what would you prefer? To keep our in-house catering services?" This is a question of food quality! (Head of primary and secondary school, Lisbon, 2011)

Despite the wider trend for the marketization of school meal services, the school management board points out how greater control over the food supplied is ensured by an in-house catering model, which they believe can also contribute to long-standing relations between children and the serving and cooking staff. Likewise, having a functioning kitchen in the school is important because it allows the kitchen staff to more easily adapt their menus to children's preferences, such as by cooking particular ethnic foods in schools situated near multicultural neighbourhoods or more cosmopolitan dishes in urban areas. However, some schools do not have the necessary cooking facilities and equipment. In these cases, the service is usually performed by catering firms wherein school meals are prepared in central kitchens responsible for providing food for several other schools sited in different localities. Meals sometimes travel several miles in thermostatic containers to their final destination. As reported by another interviewee, a dietician from a catering firm, this makes it hard to ensure that children from different schools will equally accept the same cooked dish. As she put it: 'It's 52 schools and us [central kitchen staff]. There are two thousand children who are all eating at the same time and the same thing. We notice that there are schools where they accept a particular dish better than in other schools' (Interview with a catering firm dietician, Vila Real, 2013).

In almost every school in our case studies, catering firms manage both the coffee shop and canteen services. Apart from providing food for the children, they are also responsible for hiring staff, such as cooks, serving staff and nutritionists. As reported by the school staff we interviewed, some of the more low-skilled workers are on precarious short-term contracts, with low pay, a situation aggravated by the economic crisis in the country over the past few years, putting a strain on catering firms and increasing their debts. Moreover, kitchen and serving staff can be quickly replaced after a complaint by the school about their work or malpractice within the food service. Most workers in school coffee shops and canteens are women, some belonging to immigrant and ethnic communities, with insecure and poor working conditions, including little training, low income, and few career prospects, as well working hours limited by school opening times (Fine 2005). These aspects of the work all raise difficulties for the consolidation of children's relationships with the kitchen staff, which in turn are considered to be important for 'tuning' children's tastes and for adjusting menus and food preparation in accordance to their preferences (e.g. international or regional dishes, ways of cooking and the use of local products).

Moreover, tensions and adjustments have also been identified in the management of school coffee shops and vending machines. Despite the current restrictions, some schools are unable to remove certain kinds of products due to previously-established contractual agreements made with food manufacturers and retailers. On occasion, there is pressure to keep these contracts in place, as they are important sources of income for the school:

> The problem with school coffee shops is the foods that are hard to remove: Ice-teas, sugary drinks, etc. Coca-Cola was removed. As to the vending machines, some schools have made an effort [to remove 'unhealthy' products], but teachers are not managers. There are contracts established with the vending machines franchisers and they can't get round that. And they continue to have problems with some products such as chocolate … (Representative of the Ministry of Education and Science, Lisbon, 2011)

Other schools have resisted some of the recommendations in order to enhance their surveillance over children's food choices. For example, by keeping the school coffee shop open during the lunch hour and providing particular kinds of food, the school discourages children from going out of school to buy more attractive products like hotdogs, pizzas or burgers.

Implementing food programmes and other interventions is not always an easy assignment. Some involve a high burden of paperwork for schools' internal senior managers, and the staff are not always willing to comply with this due to lack of time. Other programmes have very restrictive terms in the tender contract giving less autonomy for local producers to step in as food suppliers. Sometimes, one of the parties involved fails to comply with the established agreement, either within the local authority or the school management board. An example of this may be not offering a greater array of fruit, given the difficulty of accessing a wider variety of producers as supply is centralized and concentrated on one or two large fruit companies.

Governing children's bodies through healthy eating norms, programmes and initiatives engenders resistance and adjustment at various sites. Such processes are mediated by national and local stakeholders and conditioned by several constraints that trump an ethic of care. For instance different understandings of 'good care' (e.g. freedom of choice, health education, poverty alleviation); human resource's management policies (e.g. poor working conditions in catering firms); the availability of products (e.g. fruit variety); less-adaptable infrastructures (e.g. central kitchens); bureaucracy (e.g. rigid plans to follow and paperwork); and profit or time constraints. Although we have focused mostly on the tensions that might undermine the overall explicit aim to improve children's food practices through school meals, central and local authorities also make adjustments to enhance the acceptability of school meal biopedagogies to children, such as 'tuning' school menus to local preferences.

Embodying School Meal Biopedagogies: Acceptance, Negotiation and Rejection

School meal practices and children's bodies have become increasingly politicized spaces of intervention (Pike 2008). However, children interact with multiple contexts of consumption wherein norms and values around food nutrition and childhood are continuously negotiated and embodied (Brembeck and Johansson 2010). Even though children's experiences might be perceived as being managed by adults who take the role of 'carers', children's relationships with adults do not fully comply with the generational order that establishes both (children and adults) as socially distinct categories with marked imbalances of power. The lack of control children might seem to have in influencing, organizing and coordinating their daily practices stems from the constraints and opportunities exerted or defined by adults regarding children's ability to engage autonomously with such activities. From this perspective, childhood comprises a continuously renegotiated contract between children and adults wherein autonomy is pursued by children through challenging or simply accepting what is imposed on them. Power balances in children's relations with adults are dynamic and entail concessions or resistance from both sides (Alanen and Mayall 2001). For example, some children who had permission to leave the school premises often made autonomous food choices, such as buying snacks at the coffee shops surrounding their school or organized between themselves ways of getting access to food outside the school (see below). Moreover, although school meals consisted of a single menu with one choice of dish[3], in some cases these menus were adjusted to consider children's previous experiences with the food prepared on the menu; if a certain ingredient was repeatedly rejected by children, caterers tended to provide it less often to avoid waste.

3　Present Portuguese rules for school meals state that the single menu must consist of a soup made of fresh vegetables, one dish of meat or fish (on alternate days) and salad, brown bread, dessert (fruit, ice cream or yogurt) and water (this being the only drink allowed).

By focusing on children's agency, we take into consideration their active involvement in the negotiation of their eating habits (James et al. 2009). This perspective gives us a better understanding of the 'efficiency' and strength of school meal biopedagogies in children's bodies, as well as the tensions emerging during those processes. According to Mol et al. (2010: 10) bodies are 'unruly' elements of care that often do not submit to one's own wishes or those of carers. Thus, mobilizing care cannot be reduced to a rationalist or authoritative experience but, above all, needs to take into account a 'persistent tinkering in a world full of complex ambivalence and shifting tensions' (ibid.: 14). Thus, children continuously engage in different social, spatial and material relations affecting their bodies, senses and knowledge about food. Their food lived experiences, to cite Carolan (2011), often collide with the regulatory mechanisms designed to normalize their bodies, such as school menus.

In the focus groups conducted with children, their opinions about school meals were ambiguous and, while some criticized certain aspects of the food provided, others admitted that they were pleased with it. Most children said they did not like eating soup or vegetables, fish, and sometimes, fruit. They complained that the soup was watery, unseasoned and had visible vegetable lumps in it, that the salad was too salty or had an excess of vinegar, and that fish was served complete with bones and skin, making it difficult to eat. Some criticized foods, such as fruit, for having a rotten-looking appearance after being sliced up (i.e. oxidized apples) and burgers for their greyish colour (as they were made of turkey meat, cooked in the oven and not in a frying pan). Such critiques were usually followed by visceral reactions of disgust and repulsion, such as 'yuk' and 'bluerghhh'.

Interviewer: Do you like the food here at the canteen?

Various children: Nooooo!

Patricia: Yuk! [pulls a face]

Margarida: Now they cook loads of vegetables! And I don't like vegetables so … I eat half or almost nothing. And I eat fruit, bread and soup …

(Focus group with children, secondary school, Lisbon, 2012)

Beyond embodied and visceral displays of food rejection, children's resistance to school meals was also performed during our fieldwork in other ways. For example, piling up soup plates to hide leftovers; hiding the salad inside the bread and throwing it onto the floor underneath the table; swapping food with colleagues or even force vomiting when asked to eat foods they disliked. Still, the most common mode of resistance was simply to not eat their meals (boycotting) or to only eat the products they liked the most (food discrimination), thus leaving food behind on their trays (which eventually ended up in the waste).

We also observed children's more sophisticated strategies for avoiding adults' control over their food choices as they tried to gain access to products not available in school coffee shops. While primary school pupils are not allowed to leave school premises, those in secondary school can leave, but only with their parents' permission. Still, as observed in the playground, children do find ways to leave school or, if not, they ask others who have permission to leave to buy them food from outside. On one occasion, we witnessed several children giving money to a young girl so that she could buy them food from the retail shops outside the school. On her return she carefully passed the snacks, chocolates and sweets to the children who had ordered them through the school fence in order to avoid the security at the main gate. When we discussed this episode with the school security guard he told us that he was well aware of these 'sneaky' strategies, and that some children even profited (by asking for a small fee) from collecting food orders for others who could not leave school. Yet, he added that his hands were tied because these children had permission from their parents to go outside.

Children frequently compared school meals to their family meals, such as those cooked by their parents and grandparents, in order to establish quality standards. In almost every case, the latter were commonly perceived as the standard of good food quality. As recounted in the focus groups with children and their parents, family meals tend to accommodate family members' food preferences through a continuous and systematic daily negotiation of likes and dislikes, which can be seen as a continuous 'tinkering' (Mol et al. 2010) of careful eating practices.

> Inês: I like the taste of my mother's food better … I often say, 'Mum I'd much rather eat at home than at school'.

> Nuno: For me [the food at school] is different because at home I like the food, I think it tastes better … because I've known it since my childhood and because it's cooked by my grandmothers.

> Ricardo: I prefer homemade food mainly because of its taste.

> (Focus group with children, primary school, Lisbon, 2012)

Although school kitchen staff told us how they make an effort to prepare meals in a similar way to home cooking, the fact is that preparing dozens of meals requires different skills and experience and it is often difficult to accommodate everyone's taste. In some cases they had tried to adapt their menus by testing new flavours and removing old ones in accordance with children's preferences. They also prepared children's favourite meals on special days. Such dishes were often meat-based or inspired by national and local cuisine (e.g. grilled beef, roasts, and salted dried codfish), international dishes (e.g. lasagne, spaghetti Bolognese, pizza), fast food (e.g. chips, burgers, chicken nuggets) and ethnic foods (e.g. African curries, Chinese and Mexican food).

However, we identified differences in the ways children engaged with food across the various schools. In urban and suburban areas, these varied significantly according to the different socio-economic status of children's families. In the most affluent schools under study, children's food lived experiences consisted of regular family meals, eating out during the weekends, a few outings to fast food restaurants, tasting international cuisine while travelling to other countries, having lunch at home or in restaurants during the week, bringing snacks from home or buying them at the school coffee shops or in the surrounding area.

Interviewer: What is the strangest fruit you have ever eaten?

Frederico: It's a Brazilian fruit. It is yellow, with spikes. It's weird …

Marta: One that my mother brought from China. I don't know what it is.

Bernardo: I can't remember the name but it is a fig that has peaks and grows in cactus

(…)

Interviewer: What restaurants do you usually go to? The fast-food chains, McDonalds, pizzerias … ?

João: I go to a pizzeria that makes homemade pizzas called [says the name of a local Italian restaurant], which is close to my house but we stopped going there because once we were not served very well.

Interviewer: What about you Carlota?

Carlota: I go to [says the name of the same local Italian restaurant], it's underneath my building, and I go to McDonalds, but not often – only once a month – and whenever I go to the shopping centre.

(Focus group with children, secondary school, Lisbon, 2012)

These children often avoided having lunch at school, and when they did, it was mostly on the days in which the menu was offering their favourite dishes. In terms of their food preferences, we noticed that they varied greatly and included national and international dishes containing fish, seafood and meat, such as steak with coffee sauce, shrimps, salmon, wild-boar meat, and pizza.

In the less-affluent schools studied, the children would seldom go to restaurants. They mentioned having breakfast or buying snacks outside school more often than the affluent ones and they were also more dependent on having lunch at school. Their food preferences in turn were primarily composed of fast food, such as pizza, hamburgers and frozen lasagnes, and take-away, such as chicken. In the schools under study in predominantly rural areas, socio-economic differences were not so explicit in children's engagements with school meals. In most cases, their food preferences consisted primarily of dishes from their regions, such as meat roasts cooked at home and less frequently, international fast-food dishes such as pizza or burgers. For example, in the focus group with primary school children from a rural area close to the northern city of Vila Real, when asked whether they liked to go to McDonalds (even though a few admitted they liked it), one boy replied 'I don't like plastic food! I'm used to homemade food ... ' Regarding their acceptance of school meals, most declared they liked the food provided though they still preferred the food cooked at home. Plus, a considerable number of these children had vegetable gardens at home and their families kept animals such as cows, chickens, ducks, and horses. In these cases, children were used to playing around the animals and to helping their parents collect certain kinds of foods like eggs, aromatic herbs and vegetables.

> Interviewer: What animals do you have in your farm?
>
> Pedro: I have horses, cows, calves and a donkey.
>
> Carlos: I've got ... not horses, but ducks, chickens, pigs, dogs and cats.
>
> (Focus groups with children, primary school, Vila Real, 2012)

Despite the disciplining ambitions of regulatory mechanisms such as school meal regulations, practical adjustments emerged as almost inevitable and, in some cases, necessary to promote the acceptability of school meals. Although there are several factors influencing their degree of flexibility (e.g. school or catering firm management, staff continuity, local/central preparation of meals), adjusting procedures for food provision in schools requires negotiating with and learning from children's food lived experiences and therefore listening to their bodies. While some schools were attentive to such issues, others lacked the resources to develop solutions that match both the recommendations for healthy eating and children's preferences.

Concluding Remarks

The organization of school meals entails a wide range of practices that make it possible to mobilize care through providing food for children. By perceiving school meal biopedagogies as devices for governing children's food practices and bodies, an ethic of care implies negotiating knowledge and understandings that are produced during the exercise of 'biopower' (Wright and Harwood 2009). As we have shown, school meals' biopedagogies in their biopolitical mode often interfere with negotiations between different governmental stakeholders (e.g. central and local authorities, public officers' filing cabinets, market entities, scientific communities). Still, the ways in which carers (e.g. serving and cooking staff, teachers, nutritionists within catering firms and local municipalities) and children engage with such rules that instruct their food practices are conditioned by practical constraints and lived experiences. As a result, mobilizing care is carried out in spaces of tension where children's bodies often collide with these biopedagogies by performing resistance, rejection and adjustment through negotiation. Although some adjustments may compromise the principles of healthy eating, they are important forms of promoting acceptability and embodiment.

Moreover, by perceiving school meal practices to be innovative and creative rather than mechanically determined, we have been able to redirect our focus of analysis to the tensions and contradictions emerging from the processes of food embodied politics. As argued by Mol et al. (2010: 13) dealing with insurgent bodies and improving the efficiency of care is mostly a matter of 'practical tinkering' and 'attentive experimentation'. Care, as observed, is about negotiating institutional notions of 'good care' with children and their bodies' whims. Despite different lived experiences leading to variations in the ways in which children engage with the meals provided by schools, they are involved in a continuous process of learning and of 'becoming' where tinkering is important to mobilize an ethic of care. Thus, self-awareness and monitoring strategies should perhaps be downplayed in school meal policies. An attention to careful eating through enacting an embodied food politics should be more emphasized to establish new ways of (even if always precariously) ordering children's food practices.

References

Alanen, L. and Mayall, B. 2001. *Conceptualizing Child-Adult Relations.* London: Routledge.

Brembeck, H. and Johansson, B. 2010. Foodscapes and children's bodies. *Culture Unbound,* 2(42), 797-818.

Carolan, M.S. 2011. *Embodied Food Politics.* Farnham: Ashgate.

Carvalho, G. 2012. Health education in Portuguese schools: The contribution of the health and educations sector, in *Health Education in Context: An International Perspective on Health Education in Schools and Local Communities,* edited by N. Taylor et al. Roterdam: Sense Publishers, 37-46.

Cruz, I. 2011. Práticas de consumo: O que faz a diferença? *Sociologia Online* [online], 4, 7-25. Available at: http://revista.aps.pt/?cad=REV4e9700d167bac &autor=AUT4e97014dd28a8 [accessed: 14 May 2012].

DeVault, M. 1991. *Feeding the Family: The Social Organization of Caring as Gendered Work.* Chicago, IL: The University of Chicago Press.

European Council 2004 Regulation (EC) n. 852/2004, Official Journal of the European Union no.139. Parliament and European Council. Brussels.

Fine, M. 2005. Individualization, risk and the body: Sociology and care. *Sociology*, 41(3), 247-66.

Foucault, M. 1978. *The History of Sexuality: An Introduction*. New York: Pantheon.

Gibson, K.E. and Dempsey, S.E. 2013. Make good choices, kid: Biopolitics of children's bodies and school lunch reform in Jamie Oliver's Food Revolution. *Children's Geographies*, 11(1), 74-88.

Harwood, V. 2009. Theorizing biopedagogies, in *Biopolitics and the 'Obesity Epidemic': Governing Bodies*, edited by J. Wright and V. Harwood. New York: Routledge, 15-30.

Horta, A., Truninger, M., Alexandre, S., Teixeira, J. and Silva, V.A. 2013. Children's food meanings and eating contexts: Schools and their surroundings. *Young Consumers* 14(4), 312-20.

Jackson, P. 2009. *Changing Families, Changing Food*. London: Palgrave Macmillan.

James, A., Kjørholt, A. and Tingstaad, V. 2009. *Children, Food and Identity in Everyday Life*. Basingstoke: Palgrave.

Miller, P. and Rose, N. 2008. *Governing the Present: Administering Economic, Social and Personal Life*. Cambridge: Polity Press.

Mol, A. 2008. *The Logic of Care: Health and the Problem of Patient Choice*. London: Routledge.

Mol, A., Moser, I. and Pols, J. 2010. *Care in Practice: On Tinkering in Clinics, Homes and Farms* New London: Transaction Publishers.

Nunes de Almeida, A. 2011. *Os Nossos Dias – História da Vida Privada em Portugal* (Volume IV), Full collection directed by J. Mattoso. Lisbon: Círculo de Leitores/Temas e debates.

Pike, J. 2008. Foucault, space and primary school dining rooms. *Children's Geographies*, 6(4), 413-22.

Pimentel, I. 2001. *História das Organizações Femininas do Estado Novo*. Lisbon: Temas e debates.

Rummery, K. and Fine, M. 2012. Care: A critical review of theory, policy and practice. *Social Policy and Administration*, 46(3), 321-43.

Stoer, S.R. 1983. A reforma de Veiga Simão no ensino: Projecto de desenvolvimento social ou 'disfarce humanista'? *Análise Social*, XIX (77-78-79), 793-822.

Truninger, M., Teixeira, J., Horta, A., Aparecida, V.A. and Alexandre, S. 2013. Schools' health education in Portugal: A case study on children's relations with school meals. *Educação, sociedade e culturas*, 38, 117-33.

WHO. 2013. *Nutrition, Physical Activity and Obesity: Portugal*. Nutrition Country Profiles.

Wright, J. 2009. Biopower, biopedagogies and the obesity epidemic, in *Biopolitics and the 'Obesity Epidemic': Governing Bodies*, edited by J. Wright and V. Harwood. New York: Routledge, 1-14.

Wright, J. and Harwood, V. 2009. *Biopolitics and the 'Obesity Epidemic': Governing Bodies*. New York: Routledge.

Afterword

The Everyday Biopolitics
of Care-full Eating

Michael K. Goodman

The fascinating chapters in this book critically analyse the deeply theoretical, empirical and practical relationalities of eating, care and embodiment. As argued across the volume, multi-directional mediations among bodies, foods and caring create and are created by contingent assemblages of being in the worlds of eating. But, as the chapters also show, these relationalities are nothing if not fully political and politicized, in addition to being culturally and economically conditioned, across the scales of the personal and individual to those of the family, community, region, nation and globe. Thus, what is being spelled out in the vibrant and multi-coloured backlight of this volume is a biopolitics of the everyday: Eating and caring matter for our own and Others' fleshy bodies, whilst eating bodies transform, disrupt and co-constitute caring, not just in the multiple spaces of daily reproduction and routine, but also in those social spaces embedded with multiple ideologies and moral economies.

Caring for one's own eating body through the ingestion of food is a daily requirement as is, for many (but arguably mostly women), caring for others through the provisioning of food for children, partners, parents and friends. But so too can we now, through globalized commodity networks such as fair trade, relatively easily care for those Others and other ecologies we, in the relatively well-fed Global North, have deemed suitable to be cared for through ethical consumption. In this, ethical consumption is as much about caring for the self in drinking high quality coffee and/or eating tasty, organic meats as it is about the care for and about the Others who are able to grow and supply this quality. Yet, these requirements for quality and distinction throw up a number of biopolitical complications and borders at the heart of market-led, neoliberal forms of care-full sustainability that selectively connect us to *particular* Others and *particular* ecologies (Goodman 2013). Care, in this instance, facilitates and continues the processes of uneven development (Goodman et al. 2012).

Simultaneously, however, through global food and eating networks of the likes of fair trade, we seem to have overcome that bedevilling problem of caring about and for bodies and ecologies over spatial distance, given that ethical consumption challenges the assumption that we care most for those geographically close to us (cf. Barnett et al. 2005; Smith 1998). In essence, distance is much less of a problem for more contemporary practices of care as globalization and global connections through material and virtual means continue apace. Rather, it is *social* distance between bodies that seems much harder to overcome and which continues to bedevil. Think about it: We often avoid and step-over – both psychologically and physically – the homeless person asking for spare change outside the supermarket on our way to spend that money on a nice bag or cup of fair trade coffee. In a way, the immediacies of care can now quite easily traverse spatial distance through the immediacies of shopping for particularly 'care-full' foods. Bodies a world away are connected through fairness and care, while other closer, but perhaps more socially-distant and stigma-laden, bodies are often avoided so as to evade those more uncomfortable, bodily-present relations.

In all of this, the hunger to care for ourselves and o/Others – as mediated by the eating of food – is as much bodily and visceral as it is thought-about and chewed over; as much individualized as it is social; as much open and choice-laden as it is constrained and conditioned; as much about taste (in all its senses) as it is about access and ability. This, then, gets at what the volume's editors and several of its authors implicitly and explicitly refer to as the 'slipperiness' of the meanings, practices and outcomes of care. Defining care as slippery shines much needed intellectual light not only on care's meaningful and practical multiplicities across the foodscape, but also on how the weavings of care in, out and around eating point to its spatial and temporal contingencies. Exploring these multiplicities and the geographical and temporal contingencies of food and care is something that scholars of both foodscapes (e.g. Johnston and Goodman 2015) and 'carescapes' (Bowlby 2012) are at increasing pains to critically interrogate. Refracting these questions through the specific relationalities of eating bodies and the politics of caring, as is done in this volume, signals their conceptual and practical centrality to everyday biopolitics.

Importantly, the ways and means by which caring and eating are slippery but also made to *be* slippery points not only to these relative contingencies of food and care, but also to the ways in which they are fundamentally enmeshed with questions of power across food's carescapes. Take, as a combined example, foodbanks in the UK and foodstamps in the US. Both are seemingly provisioned under the guise of caring for the most marginal, needy and food-insecure in their respective societies, the former mostly provided by a Christian charity known as the *Trussell Trust*, the latter provided through the means-testing processes of the US Government. Statistics show that at the moment, close to a million people access and use foodbanks in the UK (Trussell Trust 2014) and the number of foodstamp recipients in the US has skyrocketed post-2008, with 50 percent of American school age children now classified as 'low income' (Southern Education Foundation 2015).

And, yet, if one were to listen to and believe the current mean-spirited chorus of conservative and right-wing pundits, commentators and politicians, these spaces and instruments of food care, however minimal they might be, are the exact opposite: For these figures, they are spaces and instruments of *un-care* that reproduce relations of dependence through the perpetuation of a culture of 'taking' without 'making' that creates 'bad' citizens, bodies and individuals. As highly visible commentators – almost none of whom have ever experienced the struggle, anger and shame of being hungry – they have worked to flip this problem on its head. As they have it, instead of providing further and greater sources of food in societies defined by recession, wage stagnation, greater tax-burdens on the poor and vastly unequal political power, care should be provisioned through the reduction of welfare payments and the demonization of foodbank clients and foodstamp recipients. Without these sources of 'free' food, these people will, therefore, 'bootstrap' themselves out of poverty, with the spectre of hunger acting as a motivational force to work that much harder for themselves and their families. The ideology and logic is thus: Taking away these 'free' goods is a form of care in the 'tough love' that motivates society's takers and skivers. So while, in these discourses and policies, un-care is positioned neatly as a form of care, the debates over food welfare have worked to demonize and exclude those with the least amongst us, confining them even further to the margins of society.

Indeed, food has historically always been at the centre of the powerful and conflicting politics of care and un-care through, for example, famines and their responses, how and by whom 'deserving' populations are defined, and who is and is not a 'good' eating citizen (e.g. Nally 2011). A more contemporary example of this is, of course, obesity, whereby the overweight are either simply dismissed or excluded as 'bad', overly fleshy citizens unable to keep their mouths shut and their bodies under control (Colls and Evans 2013). Most broadly, then, at this rather austere and insecure moment in history, we are seeing the growing expansion of a revanchist food and care politics designed for and affecting a maximum 'mean-ness' bereft of empathy or a desire to understand the daily stresses, routines or capabilities of some of society's most vulnerable citizens.

For me, the intellectual and affective inspiration to overcoming these revanchist movements is located at the centre of the two fundamental questions animated in this book: Why and how do we care about what Others eat? Posing, exploring and analysing these two questions are *themselves* a form of care about and for ourselves, for o/Others and for our wider socio-spatial worlds. They have, or at least *should* have, a normative penchant for social justice – the bigger, older brother of food justice (e.g. Cadieux and Slocum 2015; Guthman 2014; Slocum and Cadieux 2015) – at their very centre. Much beyond their robust scholarly interest, these two questions have, or again at least should have, at their core a sense of curiosity, understanding, and most importantly, empathy and compassion for the socio-economic situation of those with less than we have. These are, at their essence, *humanizing* questions about the biopolitics of the everyday that contain within them the crucial possibility of teasing out what it means to be eating, caring and embodied humans in an increasingly dour world of inequality.

But, really, *why* do we care about what Others eat? In addition to the illuminating reasons examined in this volume, I think we care because it allows us to define the similarities and differences that define who we are as individuals, as families and as communities. This question of 'why' is about both the negative and positive effects of defining members of our immediate or far-flung community, who we might bring into that community as well as what cultural and cuisine-related common ground we might or might not hold. Food, eating and caring define and bound communities of and through affect, relations and feeling. We care because this is a shorthand for who we know and should know, engage with and be around or, put in a different way, with whom we should be breaking bread. Finding, analysing and theorizing about these common culinary – and indeed, social and cultural – grounds is a critical step in pushing back against the current tide of food's revanchist cultural politics.

Drawing on some of my own contributions (e.g. Goodman 2014; Goodman in press; Goodman and Sage 2014), I feel that there are two further reasons for why we might care about eating. The first involves and orbits around body sizes and shapes. Here, we anxiously care about o/Others who are deemed too fat or too thin, that they eat too much or too little and/or that they eat the 'right' or 'wrong' foods that then sculpt their bodies in particular ways. This, of course, is tied directly to the patriarchal gaze and its processes of disciplinary 'normalization' of the female/male body. For many people, this is experienced as the troubling, socially constructed, power-laden anxieties of belonging and, literally, fitting-in through particularlized regimes of eating that are relational to caring for and about bodies.

Secondly, we seem to care about what o/Others are eating in the context of ecological health and the desire for them to do their part for the planet. Meat and products produced and shipped over long 'food-miles' have come in for a particularly bad time (cf. Sage 2012). The problem here is that, as Julie Guthman (2011) has continually pointed out, this works to overtly responsibilize consumers and their choices into *the* actors and actions that will make the planet a better place. This, of course, is something that not all of us are able to do. Indeed, here is another place where those without the means have been harangued into submission through the continuing chorus that food is *too* cheap (cf. Abbots and Coles 2013) and that saving the planet is merely a function of choice, which, of course, says nothing about costs, access and actual planetary impacts of these forms of individualized responsibilization. Thus, being unable to care through organic and more sustainable food has, too, become a kind of trope of un-care – as well as one barren of any political economic sensibilities – for those with the least among us.

Even Jamie Oliver has gotten into the act, but this time by haranguing the poor for not buying, cooking or eating healthier foods (Barnes 2015). Jamie certainly cares about what we eat – the sales of his healthy eating cookbooks notwithstanding of course! – but he does this in ways that are seemingly bereft of understanding of the experiences of those not in his circumstances. Thus, care embodied in the likes of Jamie and other, similar TV and media personalities crosses into the territory of interference (Rousseau 2012) and a powerful way through which Otherness is created, established and embedded in contemporary foodscapes (cf. Leer and Kjoer 2015).

Turning to the second question – *how* do we care about what others eat? – the obvious and most salient answer is, from my perspective, through the media and its representations of food, eating and bodies. From competitive weight-loss programmes, to competitive cooking, to the more voyeuristic shows on the struggles of obese/thin individuals, to 'freaky eaters', to the more standard documentaries, chop-and-chat shows, to those dedicated, pedagogical 'healthy eating', quick recipe cooking programmes (and related cookbooks), media content seems overtly obsessed with what, how, and why we eat the things we do. And yet, many of these how-to-cook-healthy-meals-quick shows along with the thank-goodness-I-don't-eat-that voyeuristic programmes simply get it wrong, both in terms of their moralizing as well as their practical advice (Eli and Lavis 2014). Indeed, what could be more care-*full* when cooking for someone than preparing their favourite dish regardless of health or time? And, as research shows, many poor mothers, as the primary carers and preparers of meals, tend to cook meals they know their children will eat, with concerns about health pushed firmly and frequently into the background (Bowen et al. 2014; Cairns and Johnston 2015). Feeding children foods they enjoy is a rational, adaptive strategy that works to not only ensure their children are not hungry but also, for those on a limited budget, that food does not go to waste. In a very real way, food and eating experimentation through taste innovation and development – what we are continually encouraged to do by TV shows and other food media – is now more than ever limited to the specific audiences of the 'worried-well' middle and upper-classes.

Taking this a bit further, Mike Carolan's (2011) concept of 'tuning' – deployed to describe the ways corporations have 'tuned' bodies for the tastes of industrial foods – can be re-purposed here in the context of the media, eating, caring and bodies. In short, this is a powerful idea embedded with notions of practice, embodiment and viscerality. Food media, with its growing penchant for moralization, pedagogy and boundary-making, is, thus, a powerful force in 'tuning' us to whom and what we should care about – and how to do this – across our foodscapes. Food media, whether a cooking show, a documentary or news coverage of politicians disparaging foodbank clients, is now central to the biopolitics of the everyday through its tuning of 'good' food, 'good' eaters and 'good' citizens. The follow up to this is, of course, a rather pointed set of questions: How do we *re-tune* food media to, first of all, notice socio-economic difference and take this seriously and, second, approach this difference with empathy, understanding and, as in this book, care and caring as normative means *and* ends? These are critical questions for future work around careful eating that, at least for my money, might just have food justice situated at their intellectual core.

Overall, the power of the intellectual, analytical and practical questions put forward in this book should not be underestimated. To care about and for food, care, eating and bodies is to be concerned about finding a transformative care politics and carescape, to care about people as humans with anxieties and concerns about themselves and others, as well as the multiple and conflicting understandings and practices of what food, eating and care is and should be. It is about reclaiming these revanchist food spaces back and flipping *them* on their head in the kitchen, in the cafeteria, in the restaurant, in food media and in society more broadly. Understanding and bettering the relationalities of caring, eating and bodies is central to the functioning of a just and civil society and *Careful Eating* unequivocally sets us on these critical and uncompromising pathways.

Acknowledgements

Many thanks to the editors for their very helpful comments on an earlier draft of the Afterword.

References

Abbots, E-J. and Coles, B. 2013. Horsemeat-gate: The discursive production of a neoliberal food scandal. *Food, Culture and Society*, 16(4), 535-50.

Barnett, C., Cloke, P., Clarke, N. and Malpass, A. 2005. Consuming ethics: Articulating the subjects and spaces of ethical consumption. *Antipode*, 37(1), 23-45.

Barnes, C. 2015. Mediating good food and moments of possibility with Jamie Oliver: Problematising celebrity chefs as talking labels. *Geoforum*. Available online before print.

Bowen, S., Elliot, S. and Brenton, J. 2014. The joy of cooking? *Contexts*, 13(3), 20-25.

Bowlby, S. 2012. Recognising the time–space dimensions of care: Caringscapes and carescapes. *Environment and Planning A*, 44(9), 2101-18.

Cadieux, K. and Slocum, R. 2015. What does it mean to do food justice? *Journal of Political Ecology* 22, 1-26.

Cairns, K. and Johnston. J. 2015. *Food and Femininity*. London: Bloomsbury.

Carolan, M. 2011. *Embodied Food Politics*. Aldershot: Ashgate.

Colls, R. and Evans, B. 2014. Making space for fat bodies?: A critical account of 'the obesogenic environment'. *Progress in Human Geography*, 38(6), 733-53.

Eli, K. and Lavis, A. 2014. From abject eating to abject being: Representations of obesity in 'Supersize vs. Superskinny', in *Obesity, Eating Disorders and the Media*, edited by K. Eli and S. Ulijaszek. Farnham: Ashgate, 59-72.

Goodman, D., DuPuis, E.M. and Goodman, M. 2012. *Alternative Food Networks: Knowledge, Practice and Politics*. London: Routledge.

Goodman, M. 2013. iCare capitalism?: The biopolitics of choice in a neo-liberal economy of hope. *International Political Sociology*, 7(1), 103-5.

Goodman, M. 2014. The ecologies of food power: An introduction to the environment and food book symposium. *Sociologia Ruralis*, 54(1), 94-97.

Goodman, M. In press. Food Geographies I: Relational foodscapes and the busyness of being more-than-food *Progress in Human Geography*.

Goodman, M. and Sage, C. (eds). 2014. *Food Transgressions: Making Sense of Contemporary Food Politics*. Aldershot: Ashgate.

Guthman, J. 2014. Justice to bodies? Reflections on food justice, race, and biology. *Antipode*, 46(5), 1153-71.

Guthman, J. 2011. *Weighing In: Obesity, Food Justice and the Limits of Capitalism*. Berkeley, CA: University of California Press.

Johnston, J. and Goodman, M. 2015. Spectacular Foodscapes: Food celebrities and the politics of lifestyle mediation in an age of Inequality. *Food, Culture and Society*, 18(2), 205-22.

Leer, J, and K Kjoer. 2015. Strange culinary encounters: Stranger fetishism in Jamie's Italian escape and Gordon's great escape. *Food, Culture and Society*, 18(2), 309-28.

Nally, D. 2011. The biopolitics of food provisioning. *Transactions of the Institute of British Geographers*, 36(1), 37-53.

Rousseau, S. 2012. *Food Media: Celebrity Chefs and the Politics of Everyday Interference*. London: Berg.

Sage, C. 2012. *Environment and Food*. London: Routledge.

Smith, D. 1998. How far should we care?: On the spatial scope of beneficence. *Progress in Human Geography*, 22(1), 15-38.

Slocum, R. and Cadieux, K. 2015. Notes on the practice of food justice in the U.S.: Understanding and confronting trauma and inequity. *Journal of Political Ecology* 22, 27-52.

Southern Education Foundation. 2015. A New Majority Research Bulletin: Low Income Students Now a Majority in the Nation's Public Schools [online]. Available at: http://www.southerneducation.org/Our-Strategies/Research-and-Publications/New-Majority-Diverse-Majority-Report-Series/A-New-Majority-2015-Update-Low-Income-Students-Now [accessed: 5 February, 2015].

Trussell Trust. 2014. Latest foodbank figures top 900,000: Life has got worse not better for poorest in 2013/14, and this is just the tip of the iceberg [online]. Available at: http://www.trusselltrust.org/foodbank-figures-top-900000 [accessed: 24 May, 2014].

Index

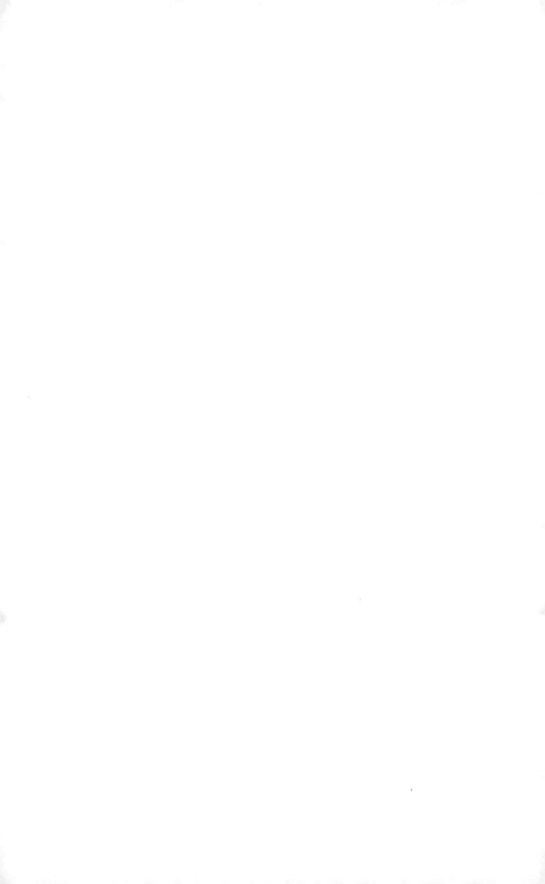

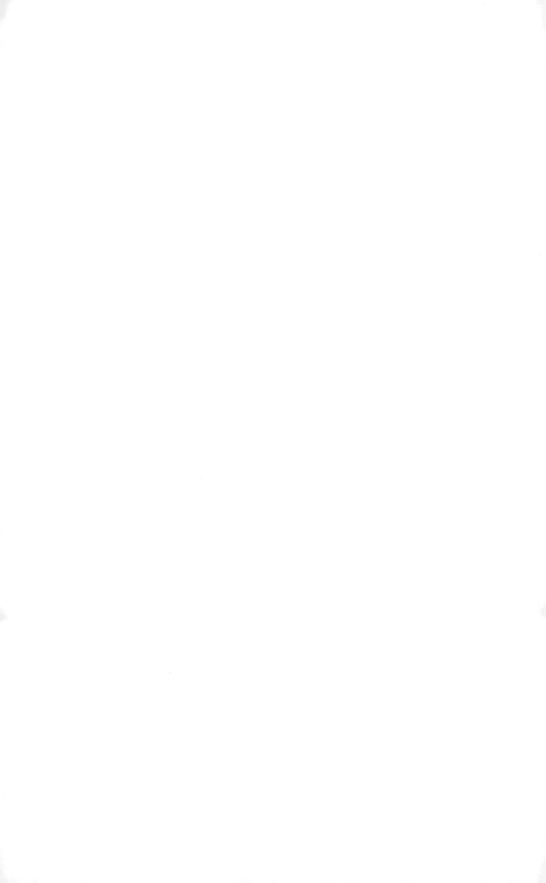

For Product Safety Concerns and Information please contact our EU
representative GPSR@taylorandfrancis.com
Taylor & Francis Verlag GmbH, Kaufingerstraße 24, 80331 München, Germany

www.ingramcontent.com/pod-product-compliance
Ingram Content Group UK Ltd.
Pitfield, Milton Keynes, MK11 3LW, UK
UKHW021002180425
457613UK00019B/784

* 9 7 8 1 1 3 8 3 0 8 4 7 3 *